in-Training
Stories from Tomorrow's Physicians

in-Training

Stories from
Tomorrow's Physicians

Peer-edited narratives written by medical students
on humanism, our real-life patients, and the
challenges of being a physician-in-training

edited by

Ajay Major & Aleena Paul

Volume 1, 2016

PAGER PUBLICATIONS, INC.
a 501c3 non-profit literary corporation

To our writers,
who have brought this compendium to fruition
with their humanity.

Contents
Volume 1, 2016

Our Patients   141

in-Training Mission Statement

in-Training is the online magazine for medical students,
founded in April 2012 by Ajay Major and Aleena Paul,
medical students at Albany Medical College.

in-Training is the agora of the medical student community,
the intellectual center for news, commentary, and the
free expression of the medical student voice.

in-Training seeks to:

enrich the medical education experience through self-reflection;

foster discourse among medical students; and

cultivate collaborative relationships between medical students
on the global stage.

Pager Publications, Inc. Mission Statement

Pager Publications, Inc. is 501c3 nonprofit literary organization
that curates and supports peer-edited publications
for the medical education community.
The organization strives to provide students and educators
with dedicated spaces for the free expression of their distinctive voices.

Pager Publications, Inc. was officially incorporated in January 2015
by its founders Ajay Major, Aleena Paul and Erica Fugger
to provide administrative and financial support for
in-Training and other publications.

in-Training
the agora of the medical student community

Ajay Major and Aleena Paul
Founders and Editors-in-Chief Emeriti

Vikas Bhatt and Joe Ladowski
Editors-in-Chief

Nina Nguyen and Andy Kadlec
Managing Editors

Editors

Phyllis Ying	Yuli Zhu	Brent Schnipke
Samantha Margulies	Claire Drom	Daniel Coleman
Mansi Sheth	Luke Fraley	Diane Brackett
Eric Donahue	Evan Torline	Angelica D'Aiello
Allison Lyle	Anne Nzuki	Natalie Wilcox
Steven Lange	Chris Deans	Tolulope Omojokun
Lindsey McDaniel	Roshini Selladurai	Chelcie Soroka
Nita Chen	Ileana Horattas	Daniel Fuchs
	Nisha Hariharan	

Nisha Pradhan
Chief Social Media Manager

Lauren Bojarski, Melanie Watt, Matthew Lenardis
Social Media Managers

Editors Emeriti

Kate Joyce	Laura Mucenski
Jarna Shah	Francis Dailey
Will Jaffee	Dragos Rezeanu
Hormuz Nicolwala	Nikki Nametz
Sanjay Salgado	Emily Lu
Jimmy Tam Huy Pham	Brent Bjornsen
Kimberly Ku	Theresa Yang
Sasha Yakhkind	Amol Utrankar

Arnold P. Gold Foundation Advisory Board

The Arnold P. Gold Foundation is a national, non-profit organization dedicated to keeping health care human. Our mission is to promote compassionate, collaborative and scientifically excellent health care and support medical trainees and clinicians so the humanistic passion that motivates them at the beginning of their education is sustained throughout their careers.

Intended to highlight the importance of humanism in medicine, *in-Training: Stories from Tomorrow's Physicians* is a unique collection of essays and poems written by medical students from across the United States. We are proud to have partnered with *in-Training* and provided grant funding to support the development of this resource guide. We are confident the personal writings and reflective questions contained here will serve as an important resource for medical students, physicians and all health care professionals.

In support of this effort, we convened an Advisory Board comprised of seasoned medical educators, clinicians, and experts in narrative medicine and writing. On behalf of *in-Training* and the Gold Foundation, we would like to thank the Advisory Board for the guidance, wisdom and feedback they provided in developing the resource guide. They each gave graciously of their time and expertise and we are indebted to their contribution not only to this effort, but to instilling the values and principles of humanism into medical education and training.

Foreword

by Richard I. Levin, MD
President and CEO of The Arnold P. Gold Foundation

While medical school is one of the most extraordinary educational experiences, it can be grueling and isolating. In the Flexner model, first year is a seemingly endless schedule of lectures, reading, research and memorization of facts. Not to mention learning a new clinical language of disease, treatments, acronyms and abbreviations. It is then followed by the clinical years marked by a dizzying dance of rounds and rotations, coupled with the simultaneous excitement of finally interacting with and caring for patients. Each year brings heightened responsibilities, more complicated experiences, persistent fatigue and longer hours. It should be no surprise then that an increasing number of medical students, even at this early stage in their professional development, report feelings of burnout and distress.

We used to practice slow medicine. Doctors (and trainees) were given nearly endless time with patients and their families to discuss symptoms, consult with peers, weigh possible diagnoses, and consider treatment options. Now, with the technological revolution and the unsustainable growth in the cost of health care, efficiency and value-based care have made fast medicine the standard. There is little time to talk to patients, let alone mentors or peers. For medical students, the current state of affairs can leave them feeling bereft of two things: time and community.

By creating this book, *in-Training* founders and editors-in-chief emeriti Ajay Major and Aleena Paul, both fourth-year medical students at Albany Medical College, have produced a resource that manages to give back a little of both. *in-Training: Stories from Tomorrow's Physicians* is an anthology of works written for and by medical students across the globe. By recruiting a dedicated group of medical students willing to write and reflect about their years in training, Major and Paul have captured the kinetic moments of medical school and provided a platform for these moments to linger online, in print, and in discussion.

A compelling aspect of *in-Training: Stories from Tomorrow's Physicians* is that it was conceived by Major and Paul before they had even started medical school. They were seniors at Union College, both involved in medical journalism, and entrepreneurial enough to want to create a platform so that they could keep writing once they started their medical studies. So, in 2012 and not yet college graduates, they started an online publication called *in-Training* that was meant to give medical students a voice and foster a community for free expression. By the time they were in medical school, they had a dedicated group of more than 40 authors submitting pieces, mainly focusing on the human side of medicine. The fact that these two editors were able to create a work of both art and science, all while under the pressure and time constraints of medical school, is remarkable. But then again, that is what many doctors do. They are often called upon to wear multiple hats — bioscientist, clinician, teacher, mechanic and nurturer.

This book represents the compilation of essays and poems published on *in-Training* over the editors' four years in medical school and reveal some of the gritty realities of medical education — from staring down your first gross anatomy "patient" to informing a living patient of a terminal disease, to performing an autopsy on a child. Some are especially harrowing, such as Ajay Koti's "Wounded Healers" about a bright, achieving med student who took her own life after years of depression.

But more often than not, the passages reflect the inner, human struggles of medical students when they are expected to express confidence yet often feel inadequate. Perhaps it is because these young trainees feel they still know so little about medicine, but feel the weight of making a correct diagnosis on their shoulders, that their vulnerability is expressed in the most human of ways, and is so easily relatable to readers.

It's not unlike Manik Aggarwal's realization in his essay, "Are There Any Physicians on Board" that just 10 days out of medical school, on a plane with a passenger short of breath, all decisions for the stranger's care at that moment were on him. Full of self-doubt, and with no one to consult, he simply had to do his best with the knowledge he had.

The format of the book itself gives nod to the themes of community and time (or the lack of each in today's health care system). Passages are short, each followed by a series of brief, reflective questions. It invites readers to take pause for a quick dose of humanity. Combining the personal accounts into common experiences that a group can reflect on creates a natural community for medical students when looking for support.

As president and CEO of The Arnold P. Gold Foundation, I am an unapologetic advocate for the need to keep health care human. Like Major and Paul, we at the Gold Foundation strive to create a community of caring — not only for medical trainees and practitioners, but for faculty, researchers, educators, and of course patients and their families. *in-Training: Stories from Tomorrow's Physicians* parallels our mission so much so that we were delighted to provide a grant to publish this collection of personal and strongly felt stories. We are confident that medical student readers — as well as other health professional trainees — will appreciate its value for helping them to preserve, sustain and nourish their humanism as they embark on what will be a difficult, exhilarating, exhausting and rewarding journey.

If this book is meant, as Major and Paul say, to be "a snapshot of what it was like to be a medical student in these four years of time," then I am encouraged. Because it means students today are reflective. They grasp the seriousness and profundity of medicine at every turn, but also have a sense of humor and a high dose of optimism. They admit their fears and short-comings, but are also confidently aware of when they have nailed it. And, most importantly, they know that compassion and empathy matter. They know that learning communication skills are just as important as learning clinical skills. And they know that taking the time to write, to express the human side of medicine, will ultimately make them better doctors. And by leaving this imprint, by offering experiences and questions to help others reflect and think, they in turn are influencing a community of future care-givers to be better doctors too.

Richard I. Levin, MD
President and CEO of The Arnold P. Gold Foundation
Emeritus Professor of Medicine, NYU and McGill Schools of Medicine

Preface

by Ajay Major and Aleena Paul
Founders and Editors-in-Chief Emeriti of *in-Training*

When we launched *in-Training* in the summer of 2012, we envisioned our fledgling publication as an *agora*, the Grecian term for the intellectual center where a community gathers to take its pulse and shape its identity. Our mission was simple: to create a virtual forum for medical students to record their thoughts about their lives as physicians-in-training. We founded the publication on two core tenets: it would be completely dedicated to the medical student community, and it would be written and edited entirely by medical students.

Within the first few months, it became clear that we had uncovered an unfilled niche within the medical student community. Wave upon wave of manuscripts rolled into our inbox: emotional stories about first patients, first joys, and first frustrations about the complexities of medicine and health care. We celebrated the honesty and courage of these narratives, written not only for catharsis and self-care, but also to offer perspective and solace in shared experiences.

Medical students craved a space for self-reflection, a space to express their innermost passions and their greatest fears about their chosen profession. *in-Training* was able to fulfill this deep-seated need, and in doing so, enrich the medical school experience by building an online community of physicians-in-training.

Having published over 850 articles by 400 medical students at hundreds of institutions around the world in the last four years, we envision *in-Training* as a written history of medical school, a living, organic document that evolves with the institution of medical education. *in-Training* is no longer a simple magazine. Impassioned opinions and authentic reflections on art, ethics, policy, literature, technology and beyond have transformed the publication into a platform for thought to turn into action, an opportunity to empower medical students to communicate with and seek support from their peers, and a place for medical students to call home.

At a time when medicine is drastically changing, we believe it is our duty to highlight medical student voices that promote the values of humanism and open discourse, and offer lessons that bolster the community. In this spirit, we present this print collection of *in-Training* pieces as a resource guide for medical students and medical educators. This compendium aims to spark self-reflection and conversations on the nature of medical education, the importance of a humanistic approach to medicine, and an appreciation for the social determinants of health.

When we selected pieces for *in-Training: Stories from Tomorrow's Physicians*, we chose narratives that represent a snapshot in time of the current cohort of medical students, their passions, and their aspirations for the future of medicine. These pieces are raw and emotional, and will resonate with students at all stages of training. Through these stories of triumphs and failings, tomorrow's physicians will be equipped to advocate for themselves, and in doing so, to advocate for the compassionate care of their patients.

We have organized the pieces into thematic sections, arranged in an order reminiscent of the milestones met by students as they journey through medical school. Of note, each piece includes the date it was originally published online. This decision was made so that readers can appreciate where each author was in their training when the piece was written, as well as to account for historical events influencing medical education at the time of publication.

While these articles were edited by our medical student editors when first published on *in-Training*, we decided against further editing when forming this collection. We wished to maintain the authenticity of the medical student voice and to highlight the mix of achievements and uncertainty that defines medical school. We avoided making retrospective changes to the pieces — while it is natural that students' opinions about specific issues will change over the course of training, we aimed to capture and preserve our writers' thoughts at that specific time in their medical school journey.

For individual medical students reading this book, we encourage you to turn to this collection whenever you wish to reflect on your experiences in medical school. Use these narratives to find lessons that you can apply to your own development into humanistic physicians. The reflection questions in this guide are written by your peers, the medical student editors at *in-Training*, and represent ideas your peers felt were necessary to their understanding and appreciation of the various decisions made during medical school. And as you move through each stage of your medical training, return to this collection to reflect how you have changed with each milestone.

For medical schools and educators, we present this compendium as a way to start conversations with your students on the key issues surrounding humanism in medicine. Whether this resource becomes part of a humanism in medicine course or a student wellness program, or a few pieces are assigned as reading before a lecture, the stories in this book will encourage reflections on the transformative experience of medical education.

For premedical students, allied health professionals, families and friends of medical students, for the patients who make everything we do worthwhile, and for anyone making decisions about the future of medicine and health care, we offer a glimpse into the personal lives and growth of your future physicians as you peruse these pages.

This collection is, at its core, a peer-to-peer guide through the transformative experience of medical school. We have embraced the premise that medical students are focused on more than just obtaining an "MD" or "DO." We recognize that medical students enter medicine with unique passions, curiosities and complexities. We hope that *in-Training: Stories from Tomorrow's*

Physicians will provide students with moments of reflection on the values that first drew them to the profession of medicine, and reaffirm their dedication to becoming humanistic physicians.

Ajay Major, MBA and Aleena Paul, MBA
Founders and Editors-in-Chief Emeriti of *in-Training*
Class of 2016 at Albany Medical College

Acknowledgements

Ingrid Allard, MD, MSEd
Joel Bartfield, MD, FACEP
James Bennett, PhD
Erica Fugger
Enid Geyer, MLS, MBA, AHIP
Elizabeth Higgins, MD
Maura Mack Hisgen
Christine M. Horigan
John Huppertz, PhD

Rebecca Keller, PhD
Kimberly Kilby, MD, MPH
Zubin Master, PhD
Mara McErlean, MD
Henry Pohl, MD
Jonathan Rosen, MD
Aviva Hope Rutkin
Carol Weisse, PhD
Melissa Zambri, JD, MBA

We dedicate this compendium to our writers, editors and readers who have made *in-Training* possible.

We thank the Albany Medical College Alumni Association and The Arnold P. Gold Foundation for their grant funding of *in-Training* and this compendium.

We thank Lynn White, MD for introducing us to the Arnold P. Gold Foundation Advisory Board who supported this book.

We would like to thank our families: Usha Vyas-Major, MD, Glenn N. Major, DVM, and Maya Major; and Paul Sebastian, Elezebeth Paul, and Merin Jose Paul.

We also wish to thank Jennifer Wilson, MS, Medical Writer and Editor at the Writing Center at Thomas Jefferson University, for copyediting this compendium.

Dissection Lab

Hands

September 25, 2013

Lisa Moore
Loyola University Chicago Stritch School of Medicine
Class of 2014

I know his hands so very well.
I get beneath the skin.
I discover what could make them tremble
Or cause the dorsum hairs to stand on end.

I intimately study these hands
That are — or, were —
Eighty-three years old.

An image is permanently burned into my mind.

I hold his hand to reposition his arm,
As if it were that of a living person.
I wonder who held it last
Before I released it from a white plastic bag.

I migrate through the lab,
Studying many bodies,
Unimpressed by faces or even genitals.
But one woman has fake nails
Painted barbie-doll pink.

No wonder we read fortunes in palms.
Those dermatoglyphs are unique indeed —
Formed in the womb,
Imprinted upon by all that we touch.

I see the living hands of my world:
Mother's precise hands, comforting with their touch
Father's wide knuckles, inherited by me
Husband's careful hands, strumming nylon strings
Grandmother's crippled hands, perfectly stroking a cat's head
Friend's talking hands, spreading their wanderlust.

These, my hands, take a scalpel and peel back the skin of another's
With the hope that one day soon these hands will heal.

Questions

1. What do you think hands symbolize in this poem?

2. Why do you think hands strike the author more than "faces or even genitals" when studying the cadavers?

3. This poem seems to serve as a catharsis for the author's experience while dissecting cadavers. Can you think of any other experiences medical students face in which poetry may help them process their emotions?

—Angelica D'Aiello

Stripping Down the Flesh: Seeing the Human in the Lifeless

February 21, 2014

Nita Chen
Albany Medical College
Class of 2017

W HEN WE PULLED BACK the crimson tarps, Mr. S did not strike me in the profound fashion I had anticipated upon witnessing a cadaver up close for the first time. After some reflecting (and a brief self-doubt as to whether I possessed sociopathic tendencies), I concluded that this was due to the acceptance that death is a very natural part of life and seeing its consequences ceased to stun me.

Having never had experienced the death of a loved one, and the fact that Mr. S was a complete stranger lying before me, made it extremely easy for me to become comfortable with his state of being. Aside from evoking the humbling gratitude of such immense sacrifice, I could not bridge the powerful connection with my "first patient" — unlike many of my fellow classmates — to experience that visceral rawness of a human being lying completely bare and under the mercy of my hands (within the boundary of reason, of course). And in some ways, I did not linger much on it other than as an obstacle in medical school that I easily (for once) passed.

Over the months and hours of chiseling away at his anatomy, I got to know Mr. S in a very intimate yet impersonal manner. I spent hours grumbling through layers of connective tissue and fat, snipping carefully away at fragile and robust fascia in the manner of an obsessive collector trying to preserve the perfect specimen, and marveling at his beautiful vasculature and nervous branches when they finally emerged. While I know nothing about who he was as a person when he was alive — his interests, his habits, his personality — I learnt that he had a really big heart (literally) and the problems that came with it, beautiful nerves and vasculature, and suffered from calcifications of his lower extremity joints.

Last week, we prepared for the nasal cavity dissection, and Mr. S's face was split in half by our professors to reveal the relevant structures. I had long stopped looking at his face just in the way we stop noticing irrelevant but constant things in our lives, but in this moment, I felt a sense of cold and cruel unstripping of someone who was once so human and — alive. Perhaps it was the time spent laboring over his body or perhaps it was just getting so used to his presence, but I felt a sadness at this necessary scene. It felt somehow inhumane, that in this practical gesture, Mr. S was no longer human but merely a — specimen.

In some ways, unknowingly to me, Mr. S had become an integral and crucial piece in my life as a medical student, and it was in viewing a face that was no longer recognizable that I really understood how real he is — and how alive he is in our minds despite having been long gone.

And perhaps, in this, I have finally found the compassion for my first patient — the one who no longer is — to color his significance in my mural of life.

Questions

1. The author describes her relationship with the cadaver as "intimate yet impersonable." How did you feel toward your cadaver during gross anatomy? How do you think we should feel towards our cadavers, and why?

2. Do you believe that we as medical students are taught or encouraged to feel a certain way towards our cadavers? Is this encouragement overt or covert? What does this suggest about the culture of medicine?

3. In some medical schools, medical students are instructed not to dissect the face until the end of the course, to prevent students from being traumatized. Do you agree or disagree with this practice, and why?

4. In this narrative, the author describes the experience of cutting the cadaver's face in half for the nasal cavity dissection. Did you have any experience in gross anatomy that you found particularly gruesome or brutal? How did you cope with it? How can medical schools prepare students for such experiences during dissection?

5. Medical students often remember most, and write the most, about their experiences in gross anatomy dissection. Why do you think this experience is so memorable or sentimental? What do you remember about your anatomy lab experience?

—Jimmy Pham

EKG Calamity
(or, Love and Cardiology)

March 18, 2014

Steven Lange
Albany Medical College
Class of 2017

In that sweet primordial pause
before knowing, before knowing you
had that brilliant *lub* without whose cause
my sinus would but sing for two.

This small sound within the chamber mocks
with flagrant range the mistook letter which
does not describe the valve but more the knock
of passion greater than mere muscle twitch.

I have no way of knowing the golden disarray:
how you would stare at tiring light
pound the heart and dry the face
to distract the paltry vagal plight.

I had a hard time charting,
partitioning my time along
the plaques and disconcerting waves,
spelling out exchanges of the veins.

An artery protrusive in the wake
of normality overflown
swells in the quake of giving up
elastic chance to liquid throes.

A sudden meeting of a pulse becomes
null reverberations of the sternum:

the shared plate where sullen sinks
trace the face of this predicament.

The studded wall of your vibration
forms a constellation where the halls
of rogue eddies and emancipations
of excited bursts bear my many falls.

The tonic fire now subsides,
settles in the wash of flooded rooms
while your love lately follows the news
and lavishes in atrial blues.

I would be shocked to find the spout
of piping choking up with lust
coating the underside of coughs
and filling up the air with mitral doubt.

Your walk denies the hypertensive drive
of ventricles adapted to defeat
and though we seldom find our love alive
your dear resistance served its every beat.

Questions

1. In the pair of pieces by this author, EKG Calamity and M/R/G (page 186), the author describes well-functioning and failing hearts. Discuss how the author highlighted aspects of patients' lives by focusing on their hearts. What imagery does the author use to showcase health and to portray disease?

2. In one piece, the author focuses on the anatomy of the heart; in the other, the author places the heart in the context of the suffering patient. How do you think your perception of anatomy will change or has changed from gross anatomy dissection to real patients? Is this perceptual change important?

3. In both poems, the author interlaces rich emotional language into the heart's repetitive physiology. What emotions did you feel during gross anatomy dissection? How were those emotions similar to or different from the emotions you feel when treating patients?

—Aleena Paul

Lacrimosa

July 13, 2014

Daniel Coleman
Georgetown University School of Medicine
Class of 2017

I STARED AT HER REMAINS, all of the little bits and pieces. It was the last day of gross anatomy and I wanted the moment to feel important. I wanted Her to know what it had meant. The sacrifice. As we zipped up the Tyvek bag, I wanted Her to hear angelic voices and heavenly bells. It was what She deserved; it was what they all deserved. To hear John Taverner when we placed her into the box, a Magnificat so thick and lofty you could almost see the sound shimmer in the air. To hear inspiration and hope as we closed the lid, just before everything became silence.

I didn't hear any of that, and I was halfway home before I realized that I had never even prayed for Her.

I used to think that death was a rare thing because I didn't know anyone who had died. It was abstract and unreal, something that happened in movies to make adults cry. I thought that death was a rare thing until I was eight. That was when Angela Pollock died of cancer. She was the wife of a family friend; someone we would see around Christmas or maybe at a summer barbecue. When I think of her now, I see her picture on the prayer card. Thick-rimmed glasses and a red sweater. I'm pretty sure she was smiling. There were a lot of people at her funeral, and I remember thinking that it must be nice to have so many people be sad you were gone. I didn't even know that many people. Afterwards, my parents told me to pray for her, so I did.

I had a poster on the wall of my room. It was a picture of an astronaut during spacewalk, tethered to his ship by nothing more than a thin, white gossamer. It all seemed so delicate. I wondered what would happen if the filament broke and he just disappeared. In bed, I would stare up at the poster and say an *Our Father* and a *Hail Mary* and a *Glory Be*. And then I prayed for Mrs. Pollock, that she wasn't scared, that she was somewhere good. I would make the sign of the cross and say an amen. On most nights I fell asleep before I could finish, and would suddenly find myself dreaming of great things, like flying over the ocean, always towards the sun as it sank into the fold of night.

I liked praying for Mrs. Pollock because it felt important, like I was helping in some unknowable way. So it wasn't long before I decided to start praying for everyone who died, even those I didn't know. I would watch the news and pray for the victims of that fire or the couple who was killed across town. There was a man two streets over who died of a heart attack in his house, so I prayed for him, too. The Priest always had a few new names at Sunday Mass, and I would add my prayers to his. There was even the bird that flew in front of my brother's car, meeting its maker in a most glorious burst of blue plumage. I wasn't sure if there was a Heaven for birds, but I prayed for it anyway. I imagined my words were like bits of cloud beneath this great collection of souls, dissolving their earthly bonds, propelling them forward, forever into the sky.

And then my Aunt Andrea passed. Luke got hit by a car. Frank overdosed on cocaine. Father George. Steve. Johnny. Nana. Grandma. By the time I was 27, I was no longer a stranger to death. It wasn't an everyday occurrence, but it certainly seemed to happen a lot to people I loved.

"People die. That's what happens when you get older."

That's what my uncle said after my Grandma's funeral. He said it in such a casual, off-hand way, but I remember thinking he was right. Death no longer felt rare or important and, eventually, I decided there were only so many souls a prayer could lift. At some point, I just stopped praying.

Five years later, I met Her in gross anatomy. Running my fingers over the grey, compact skin, I wondered if She knew it would be this way. Puncture wounds in Her neck and leg, embalmed blood congealed in Her veins. Maybe She just didn't care. It was easy to think that way. It made things easy. Initially, the process felt very removed. We skinned Her arms and legs, carefully digging through the layers of tissue to identify the clinically relevant structures. We settled into the routine of seeing Her a few times a week, and indeed, we became fair friends with death.

Then, just before Christmas, I held Her heart in my hands. We had just cut a flap into the right atrium, and I peeled back the wall, staring into the depths of that great machine, so small and delicate. I was awed, honored, realizing for the first time the extent of Her sacrifice. She had given herself over to untrained, clumsy hands so we might someday become doctors and surgeons and heroes. It must have taken so much courage to allow this to happen, to continue existing in this way long after her last moment. I wondered if I had that courage. It would only be right, in a twisted, Golden Rule type of way. Do unto yourself as you have done to others. But I don't know, even now. Because what if She was still there, Her mind or Her soul, feeling everything, painfully waiting to be liberated? It was a horrifying thought that made the significance of Her death all the more evident. Some wise person had told us that She would be our first patient and our greatest teacher, but She was more, even than that. We had to set Her free.

So we dug carefully through the thin white webs of intervening fascia, watching them dissolve into thin air. We demonstrated the paths of Her vessels and nerves, hewn out of the surrounding tissue. We categorically identified every structure we could, even removing the lungs, bowels, and brain for deeper inspection. We were like the ancient Egyptians, sending Her soul piece by piece into the afterlife. At the end, I was left staring at Her remains, all those little bits and pieces we placed so neatly in a box, hoping She knew what it meant.

Lying in bed that night, I said an *Our Father* and a *Hail Mary* and a *Glory Be*. And then I prayed for Her. Not a prayer of hope, but one of thanks.

I wasn't wrong. Death really is a rare thing. It is a single moment among all those other moments of our lives. It is the last moment. When it comes to me, I hope I can pass through the gate with courage. I hope to hear angelic voices and heavenly bells. To find myself flying over the ocean towards the sun as it sinks into the fold of night, buoyed by the thoughts of those I left behind. I hope that somewhere, a child prays for me just before he falls asleep and goes on to dream of great things.

Questions

1. How has your medical school experience changed your perception of death, if at all?

2. How do you (or do you think others) reconcile the scientific need of "seeing to believe" with religious devotion? How will you manage these issues with your patients in the future?

3. Why do you think the author capitalizes the pronouns "Her" and "She" throughout the piece?

4. Why do you think people donate their bodies to the "untrained, clumsy hands" of medical students?

—Daniel Coleman

autumn autopsy

September 10, 2014

Abi Ashcraft
Medical College of Wisconsin
Class of 2015

as I walk away from your linoleum tomb
I run my tongue over cracked lips
for the first time
and they are no longer attached but
hanging
like you were and will always be
suspended from cold mental concrete
waiting
for warm hands to pull you down and then
pull you apart
before your body bursts into a thousand crisp autumn leaves
and the wind scoops you up
scatters beautiful bright sun droplets over your veins and facets
and gently lies you down in a black plastic bag
at the curb at dusk

Questions

In this brief and poignant poem, the author paints a scene that suggests
the memorial ceremony that many medical schools have for their cadaver
donors. What was your memorial ceremony like? What emotions did you
feel, and did it change the way you felt about your cadaver? Were you able
to meet family or friends of your cadaver? If so, how did you feel about that
experience? If not, would you have liked to meet them? Why or why not?

—Ajay Major

A Tub of Baby Hearts

September 22, 2014

Katie Taylor
Icahn School of Medicine at Mount Sinai
Class of 2016

THE PATHOLOGIST IS DOLING OUT defective baby hearts from a dripping plastic tub. A few drops splash onto the student next to me. The pathologist claims it is just water. Water, and dead baby heart juice, that is. All of these baby hearts have congenital defects, and the ones we hold now each have a ventricular septal defect, a big hole in the middle of their heart that killed them. We have been allotted fifteen minutes to study these hearts. The gray mush I hold in my purple, latex-gloved hand looks like a little hummingbird heart; it's the littlest heart I've ever seen, no bigger than my thumb. It takes a while to orient myself around this tiny organ, which has been pre-sliced into thirds to reveal the insides of the ventricles and atria. Attached to my heart are two floppy, spongy lungs, and six inches of aorta, which has been sliced open and splayed flat to reveal its astoundingly smooth interior. In the middle of that tiny heart, indeed we find a tiny hole. The timer rings, our fifteen minutes are up.

We plop our hearts into the tub and pass it along to the group next to ours. We are delivered a new tub of soaking baby hearts, this bunch all with transpositions of the great vessels. Instead of the big aorta coming off of the sturdy left ventricle, the wimpy pulmonary arteries have sprouted instead. The heart I hold has an intact umbilical artery and vein, which run to and from the neonatal heart. At the end of those vessels there hangs a circle of skin, this dead baby's severed belly button. This skin that once connected mother to child. This skin that the mother perhaps stroked while her baby lived. And maybe still stroked after it died. I am astonished by how skin-like it is. It looks like my skin.

In addition to a bellybutton, this dead baby heart came with a small plastic tag that hangs by a soggy white string. Like a toe tag. It turns out this baby died in 1972. In fact, the pathologist tells us, all the baby hearts are from the

70s. Advanced technology has allowed women to learn much earlier in their pregnancy of possible fetal heart anomalies. If one is discovered, and there is no cure, many women abort. If the faulty heart is fixable, new life-saving surgeries have allowed most of the defective-hearted infants of today to grow into adolescence and adulthood.

These babies from the 70s, however, were not so lucky. Their hearts have since far outlived their bodies. Exhibited for decades now, they are taken from their sopping tubs for two hours of scrutiny and fame during our medical school's annual congenital heart defect day.

The ashen heart in my hands pumped probably for only a few minutes, the pathologist explains. With the great vessels transposed, oxygenated blood cycles to the lungs, then back to the left heart, then back to the lungs, in parallel with but never to the rest of the body. All the other tissues died a hypoxic death. Timer rings. Next tub arrives.

Questions

1. This narrative mentions new technologies that have been put into practice. In the age of increasing medical advancements, do the older methods of teaching still have a place in medical education, or should they evolve as well?

2. The piece, much like the baby hearts the author describes, dies abruptly. What emotions do the author's descriptions stir?

—Allison Lyle

Autopsy of a Child

January 27, 2015

Erin Baumgartner
University of Louisville School of Medicine
Class of 2016

It's a brief coming-going ghostly meeting.
The tiny form bereft of life so fleeting.
Eyes, like thin rings of stone, two
dry pomegranates, parched black dew.
So still, with a soul fixed colder,
untimely severed ne'er fading older.
Grieved, naïve, yet seeming wise,
the ash-sad dusty doll vacant lies
with mimic-mien, and quickened guise.
A scalpel-split red reading frame
seeps voices quickly smothered, slain.
Probing for a tale at doubt's behest,
with hope-dread, for foul or fair witness.
But either grim reply fails those who mourn
Lifting lightly the anguish-burden borne.

Questions

1. Physicians-in-training are often exposed to experiences far outside of their comfort zone, like the author's observation of a child's autopsy. What jarring experiences have you had to cope with in medical school? How did you cope with them? In the future, how would you work to keep yourself from becoming too detached, while maintaining your equilibrium in the face of such difficulty?

2. The author forms a bond with the deceased in a short period of time. Is this a defense mechanism, or something more?

3. The death of a child seems unfair and unjust. An autopsy of a child seems violent and unimaginable. If you were the one wielding the scalpel, would it be any different than an adult cadaver dissection?

—Allison Lyle

Anatomical Variation

February 3, 2015

Damien Zreibe
University of South Florida Morsani College of Medicine
Class of 2018

Utmost respect to the admirable ones,
who gave us their bodies to cut,
peace to their souls as I dissect their soles,
their heart, their lungs and their gut.

I wish I could learn from this body of bones,
and muscles and nerves and veins,
but to me it's a sea of fixed tissue and fat,
and worries and stresses and pains.

All the muscles are stuck and have fused into one,
all the veins are embedded in fat,
less time is spent learning and more in worrying
if it is this I should cut, or it is that.

I never know if I'm deep enough,
and I'll sever a nerve, maybe six,
not that it mattered, I couldn't tell them apart,
I'm just hoping some material sticks.

Nothing ever looks the way that it "should,"
and guessing never helped me learn,
so I stand on the side with my scalpel in hand,
hoping they don't give me my turn.

'Cause it always looks different and never works out,
never matches the pro-section...
and the professor just shrugs, unhelpful as ever,
"Anatomical variation."

Questions

1. How does the playful meter of the poem highlight or distract from the stark and often uncomfortable reality of the once-living patient?

2. How does anatomical variation complicate medical education? How does it affect our understanding of the human condition?

3. At the end of the poem, the author implies that the methods for teaching gross anatomy don't match the needs of the learner. Have you encountered this problem in medical school? What did you do about it? What do you think institutions can do to prevent this disconnect in their students?

—Steven Lange

Hello Sir

March 19, 2015

Haikoo Shah
Northeast Ohio Medical University
Class of 2018

HELLO SIR,
I didn't think this would be an apology letter. But it is.

When I opened up the gurney for the first time, I expected to be overcome with this profound, epiphanic wave of emotion. I thought this would be one of those slow motion, cinematic, defining moments in my training. I thought I would be solemn. I thought I would be grateful. I thought I would be curious. I wasn't.

You were overweight.

I could see the smooth rolls of skin around your sides, around your neck, around your arms. I could see your stomach underneath you, like a balloon being pressed under the weight of your coarse, wide back. I could see the hours that we would spend peeling layer after layer of fat off you.

I lost any sort of avidity that comes with being a fresh-faced student. This was going to be a long semester.

Three days a week, we would come into lab, spend a few hours removing fat from your body and leave without finding 70 percent of the structures we were supposed to. At first, we would try to find some of the nerves and blood vessels embedded in your fat. At first, we were careful about leaving as much skin intact as possible. At first, we cared.

As the semester went on, all that quickly disappeared. Our cuts become coarser and deeper. Your body became smaller and smaller. Our frustration became louder and crasser.

We weren't learning anything from you. The adipose permeated every inch of your body, making even large muscles indiscernible. The nerves and arteries were the same color of the adipose; as we cut away the fat, we'd inadvertently cut away all the neurovasculature. Your fat oozed a milky liquid, so much liquid that it formed a pool around your body with bits of fat globules and pieces of skin floating around. It was awful. It was frustrating. It was a waste of time.

And then we got to your lungs.

Covered by metastases, so many metastases. Small, hard black nodules pervading your smooth pink-tinted lung tissue. One by one, these small tumors had spread through your body and had grown, carelessly destroying the surrounding tissue.

The wave that I was expecting earlier came now and in a different form. It was no cinematic epiphany. It was a slow, sobering realization. A realization of how quickly we can lose our humanity. I looked at your body and I didn't feel anything. I did not see a human body lying in front of me. I saw muscles. I saw skin. I saw adipose.

I saw how erringly easy it is to lose yourself.

You did not teach me the human anatomy. You showed me something far greater.

I'm sorry.

Thank you.

Questions

1. Were there times during your training when you were concerned about losing your humanity? How did you react, and how did you work to bolster and maintain your humanity in the aftermath?

2. The author writes this narrative as an apology letter. Is there anyone to whom you feel you to need to write an apology letter? A patient, a family member, a colleague? What would the letter say?

—Aleena Paul

Learning Curve

I Don't Know:
The Medical Student Motto

September 29, 2013

Daniel Lefler
Cooper Medical School of Rowan University
Class of 2016

IT TOOK ONE DAY of medical school to kick me off the high horse I rode through the months leading up to it.

"Repeat after me," said one of our administrators as he quieted down the eager students. "I am a first-year, and I know nothing. Remember that."

It was completely true. (A year later, it probably still is.) To all of my family members who keep asking me what that rash is: I don't know. To all of my friends from college who ask me if they can still drink while on a certain medication: the answer is probably no, but I have no idea. And finally, to my parents who asked if something my dog swallowed would kill her: I am not in veterinary school.

Since the day I was accepted into medical school, the people around me suddenly saw me as a doctor with a vast pool of knowledge. Perhaps my friends and family were too supportive to know enough to doubt me, but I have no doubt that other medical students experience much the same thing.

A year later, I have some knowledge. To be honest, I occasionally recognize something from my studies or something that I have seen in clinic. In those cases, I have to calm myself down at the idea that I actually know something useful. I still do not know enough to diagnose a patient properly or to give the right answer when someone asks me a medical question. I might be able to help my brother buy the right over-the-counter cream for that rash on his arm.

In short, that makes me only slightly more qualified to disperse health care advice than a neurotic mother using WebMD.

My lack of knowledge does not stop people from asking me for advice, though, and I wouldn't have it any other way. Every question is an opportunity to apply the facts I learn every day to something real, or to look up the answer and learn it that way. I am never afraid to say "I don't know" in those

25

situations, and I hope that never changes.

I hope what *does* change is the frequency with which I say it. Every question that is asked of me is one that I will ask someone with more experience who can teach me the answer. With time, I will never have to say "I don't know" to the same question twice.

The reason that we go into the field of medicine is that we like being constantly challenged by questions. We like the process of finding the answers, and we want to be able to apply our knowledge to a good cause. Part of our development is having enough confidence in ourselves to say "I don't know."

And there's nothing wrong with that.

Questions

1. The author of this narrative speaks of family and friends who are "too supportive to know enough to doubt" him. Have you had an opposite experience, perhaps a family member who is a physician, who has criticized you for not knowing something? How would you react to that criticism?

2. How do you cope with the vast quantity of information that you are expected to know? Is it humbling, frustrating, or motivating to always be learning? Is it something else?

3. What do you think of the "I know nothing" motto that the administrator made the students recite? Was that appropriate or too harsh?

—Diane Brackett

Medicine's Hardest Lesson: People, Not Patients

October 28, 2013

Navdeep Kang
George Washington University School of Medicine
Class of 2015

MEDICINE IS DIFFICULT. It's not that the road starts years in advance of medical school, taking difficult premedical courses, volunteering at hospitals or emergency services. It's not the notorious competition and stress of simply being accepted to training. It's not the life-consuming monster of training itself.

The difficulty of medicine is people. If you immediately thought of our patients, perhaps that's the problem. Our patients are the easiest part of medicine. We sit down at rounds, we create an addressable list of problems to objectify and quantify a patient's — and hardly ever do we say "person's," — story.

People and persons can be easily lost in medicine. To begin, we can start with the most obvious example, our patient. A person becomes a patient the moment they see a doctor. The doctor listens attentively, analyzing and organizing a patient's story to the set algorithm of the history of present illness, past medical and surgical histories, medications and allergies, assessments and plans. By the end of the visit, if there is still a person behind the patient, it becomes neatly organized and filed under "Social History," which all too often is nothing more than objective occupational, travel and dietary data.

It's a cold framework, but it's the framework which powers our clinical duties. It's the structure which allows us to best deliver care and medicine, without subjective skew. For decades of professional practice, 8 to 14 hours a day, it will dominate our every interaction with every new stranger in clinic. And this, however, says nothing of the years spent purposefully and diligently ingraining this mentality into our psyche, facilitating that transition from procedural recollection to habit.

This is precisely the problem, the difficulty of medicine. Cool analytic thought is intentionally drilled into habit. Habit lets you instantly, seamlessly, swiftly slip into practiced routine. Habit stays with you. But habit does not run by the clock. Habit, by nature, is always on.

That's the hardest lesson of medical school. Our training sculpts us and shapes us, but it isn't something that we simply leave in our white coat when we go home. Perhaps this is what is meant by "medicine is a way of life." Learning that our training shapes us, as people, and what that means for the people in our lives, is hard. It isn't because it's hard to observe. It's because it's a hard truth to face.

Tireless work ethic, dedication, objectivity, selflessness and selfless compassion: qualities that define an excellent physician. But do they define an excellent friend? Do they define an excellent spouse? Desirable qualities to be sure, but most might say no. Physicians have divorce rates 10 to 20 percent higher than the national averages, and of marriages that stay together, they're less happy. Physicians are at greater risk of depression, as high as 30 percent among newly-minted interns. Most troubling of all, physician suicide rates are more than double the national average. The void left behind each year is large enough to be filled by one or two entire medical school classes.

Scary. Frightening. Sobering, to be sure. But lessons must be learned. Without an understanding of the reality we face, however cold and cruel that might be, we cannot hope to overcome it. If our medical training teaches us anything, it is that through knowledge, understanding and dedication, the scariest demons become manageable, even conquerable. Understanding what we face helps us prepare. It becomes easier to remember to stay balanced. It becomes easier to remind ourselves of the person behind the patient. Our spark, our creativity, the things that make us human are harder to forget when we know their value. In that sense, the hardest and starkest lesson of medical school becomes a blessing. The hardest lesson of medical school becomes an opportunity to develop a rare wisdom. It's that wisdom which makes us, less importantly, better doctors. It's that wisdom which makes us, more importantly, better people.

Editor's note: On August 27, 2014, Navdeep Kang died in a motorcycle accident in Maryland. He was a fourth-year medical student at the George Washington University School of Medicine. We hope this article allows Navdeep's legacy to live on as part of in-Training and the medical student community.

Questions

1. Does being a good doctor make you a good person? Do you think medicine changes who you are as a person? Why or why not?

2. How do you think physicians strike a balance between analytical thought and emotive thought when interacting with patients? How do you envision yourself striking that balance in your own practice?

3. The author mentions the importance of qualities that allow us to form strong relationships in our personal lives, such as with friends and spouses. How do these qualities impact the physician-patient relationship, if at all?

—Phyllis Ying

Searching for Role Models in Medicine: Where Have All the Giants Gone?

February 7, 2014

David Gasalberti
Drexel University College of Medicine
Class of 2015

THROUGHOUT MY ROTATIONS, I often wondered what it must have been like to train under the tutelage of Michael DeBakey, a pioneer in cardiac surgery, or Harvey Cushing, the father of modern neurosurgery. I imagined myself scrutinizing a CT scan (or a plain x-ray in Cushing's time), having these masters of medicine critique my differential diagnosis or being in the operating theater learning a new operative technique. I tried to imagine the immense satisfaction one must have felt to have their approval or even praise.

During my surgical rotation, I distinctly remember my attendings regaling us with stories from their days as newly minted residents and their interactions with the giants of their time. Aside from the frequent mythologizing that seemed to accompany every story, occasionally a pearl or two of wisdom would be yielded and I would walk away from the conversation wondering who and where are these great physicians in my time.

Are they confined to the hallowed halls of Massachusetts General Hospital or the Mayo Clinic? Are they an endangered species relegated to the ivory towers of American medical education? As my rotation drew to a close, I was distraught by the fact I could not name an attending or resident that I wanted to emulate with any serious conviction. Perhaps I had set the bar slightly out of reach.

I was rotating at a small community hospital known more for its works of charity than its commitment to the advancement of medicine. I realize that how one defines a giant in any field is entirely subjective and that my examples above emphasize certain qualities: a commitment to medical advancements and a penchant for thinking outside of the box. In retrospect however, I may have been too restrictive with who I viewed as a giant.

Every day at this community hospital, I cared for some of the most vulnerable members of our population: the poor and uninsured. I recall one patient with severe sleep apnea requiring a tonsillectomy. He had been turned away by five other surgeons before ending up in my mentor's office. The patient had myriad other medical problems in addition to being uninsured.

When I asked my mentor why he decided to proceed with the surgery he replied: "This patient has been kicked around the medical system for far too long. Maybe it's the idealist in me but the buck needs to stop somewhere." His comments rekindled the idealism I once had upon entering medical school. Not a day went by on the surgical service when I did not encounter a similar situation: a patient on the fringes of the medical system finally crossing paths with doctors willing to put the patient's interests ahead of their own despite the liabilities.

As I continued to reflect, I realized that my laughably narrow definition of a great physician, a "giant," needed broadening. While the mentors I had may not have been the forerunners in their field, they exemplified the virtues of compassion, sacrifice and humility that the field of medicine always requires. The unsung acts of humanity that unfolded before my eyes every day in clinic made them great physicians. I had indeed walked among giants.

Questions

1. How has medicine changed since the days of Cushing or DeBakey? Do you feel this is why there are fewer "giants" in the field?

2. What makes a person a strong mentor or "giant"?

3. What are the "giants" at your medical school or hospital doing that makes them noteworthy, and how can you set yourself up to follow them?

4. What qualities do you look for in a mentor? Do you currently have a mentor? What is your relationship with that person like? Do you consider that person a "giant"? If you do not have a mentor, where can you go to ask for help finding one?

—Joe Ladowski

It's Hard Keeping a White Coat Clean

October 27, 2014

Claire McDaniel
Georgetown University School of Medicine
Class of 2018

As I WAS STANDING in my apartment building's laundry room scrubbing away at a stubborn coffee stain, I kept up a steady stream of curses at my white coat. In the seven weeks since I'd first donned it, my coat had apparently decided that it preferred to be any color but white. A Tide-to-Go pen is now a permanent fixture in my pocket, and it's used almost as often as the actual pens.

It's odd how much can be invested in a single article of clothing. The white coat is supposed to be a testament to clinical respect and cleanliness, coffee stains not withstanding. It acts as the uniform of our profession, an unofficial signal to other physicians and medical students that we are kith and kin. It certainly helps perpetuate our own beliefs that we are the white knights, riding into battle against disease and suffering.

Somehow, though, I feel like an impostor when I wear it. I'm a first-year medical student, besieged by biochemical cascades. What do I know of the responsibilities of truly wearing the white coat?

Every time I have put on my coat and gone into the hospital, I have been asked for directions, been given priority for getting on elevators or other small acts of respect. Frankly, I don't feel like I've earned that respect. Not yet, anyways.

First-year medical students like myself have barely dipped our toes in the waters of medicine. Attendings ask me what tests I would like to order for a theoretical patient, and all I can do is stare blankly at them and mumble something I heard once on an episode of "E.R." We simply don't know enough to be able to answer most medical questions. If you want to know about adrenal cortex hormones or diabetes, though, I'm your gal.

I might not know a lot yet, and studying every day is exhausting. But when I trudge home from the library after learning an endless series of enzymes that all manage to sound the same, I see my white coat in my closet. It's a symbol of perseverance, a reminder that I — and my fellow students — took an oath to which we must adhere for the rest of our lives.

The coat is a symbol of responsibility, binding us into the roles we swore to fulfill — healer, advocate and student. Perhaps we don't know enough to treat patients (spoiler: we don't), but the coat is a promise that we will, a promise that we will strive to deserve the respect with which it invests us.

Standing on stage at my white coat ceremony, I wasn't aware of that promise. I was too giddy to think that far ahead. Along with the thoughts of "Can my parents see me?" and "Don't trip!" that were running through my mind, there was still a sense that something larger was being bestowed, something more important than a boxy white cotton coat.

We were told when we first put on our coats that we were entering the medical profession. They just didn't mention that, for better or for worse, we were being pushed in the deep end and told to swim. Don't get me wrong, I am elated at the trust that is being placed in us. However, it places the onus on us to live up to that respect. And *that* is the true power of the white coat.

Questions

1. What does the white coat symbolize to you? Is it a garment of respect, or a disgusting fomite? How does this differ from what it symbolizes to patients and their families?

2. Do you feel that wearing your white coat helps or hurts your rapport with patients? Why?

3. Have you had any memorable encounters that occurred solely because you were wearing your white coat?

4. Like the author, did you ever feel like an "imposter" in your white coat?

—Nikki Nametz Feinberg

Medical Student, Student Physician or Student Doctor?

January 13, 2015

Joshua Niforatos
Cleveland Clinic Lerner College of Medicine
Class of 2019

A FTER INTRODUCING MYSELF as a first-year medical student working with the attending physician, I went through the medical history with the patient to ascertain his chief complaint and the history of present illness. Since this was only a six-month follow-up appointment in an internal medicine outpatient clinic, there was not much to cover besides checking whether his medications were up-to-date and how he had been managing his chronic conditions. As this was my last patient of the day, I asked if I could practice various aspects of the physical exam that were not necessary for his appointment. Typical of my experience in longitudinal clinic, the patient obliged and thought it was great that he would get some "additional care."

"Are you a fellow or something?" he asked during the exam.

"No, no. I'm a first-year medical student," I reminded him.

It seems that "fellow" and "medical student" were synonymous to this individual.

Part of the curriculum of my medical school includes various readings in both the social sciences and the humanities. We recently reflected upon the titles we are known by, such as medical student, student physician or student doctor. More specifically, what is meant by the names and titles we are known by? After contemplating how to introduce myself to patients, I offer the following reflection.

Renowned sociologist Erving Goffman popularized the notion that "the self" is a performance based on a culturally-constructed script.[1] This script, according to Goffman, is composed of "performers and audiences; of routines and parts; or performances coming off or falling flat; of cues, stage settings and backstage; of dramaturgical needs, dramaturgical skills, and dramaturgical strategies." The medical student and patient encounter is a *performative* moment in which both the student and the patient play dual roles as performers and audience members. This idea of performance is further complicated by Chicago sociologist Robert Ezra Park's comments in "Race and Culture": "It is probably no mere historical accident that the word person, in its first meaning, is a mask. It is rather a recognition of the fact that everyone is always and everywhere, more or less consciously, playing a role."[2]

The idea that the medical student is playing a role influences how I introduce myself to patients in longitudinal clinic. Before attending medical school, I assumed various titles, including college student, graduate student, seminarian, theology student, pre-med, anthropology student, biology student and social scientist. I use these titles, or script *identifiers*, to answer questions like "what do you do?" or "what do you study?" Stated another way, I use "script" terms that are easily identifiable to others within my culture despite the fact that these terms have little existential significance for me. Rather than providing a long monologue on who I am and what I study, I wear a mask and put on a show in order to engage in quick and effective communication. When I am taking a medical history and going through the physical exam, I am at once a performer of the art of medicine for the patient, as well as an audience member to the performance and narration of the patient's illness.[3]

So, how do I introduce myself to patients in clinic? I have chosen to identify myself as "a medical student working with [the attending physician]." In our society, patients are more likely to know what "medical student" means compared to "student physician" or "student doctor." However, my longitudinal clinic experience seems to indicate that patients are often unaware of what is meant by the term "medical student." Thus, one should proceed with great caution when determining how to identify him or herself to a patient.

Marracino and Orr state that "the patient could expect a responsible learner who performs what he is trained to do under the direct and constant direction of a licensed doctor. This approach is in accord with moral and legal principles — a solution that fulfills ethical duties to the patient and provides an optimal environment for learning."[4] If the goal of medicine is to learn how to heal and cure patients, as well as accompany them on their journeys of illness and flourishing, then establishing an honest relationship with the patient is of utmost importance.[5]

A critical analysis of the ethics of medical student performance and its role in obtaining an illness narrative from the patient has yet to be written. Will a medical student receive different information from the patient depending on the name she uses to introduce herself? Is a patient more likely to divulge the details of her illness if she thinks the student in front of her is a fellow as opposed to a medical student? Is the goal of medicine solely to ascertain the health concerns of the patient in order to implement a plan to address these concerns, like a technician? I push back and ask: should not the way information is obtained, specifically in the context of the patient's perception of the performer in front of her, be considered carefully in order to avoid the dangers of medical paternalism?

At the end of the day and ethical considerations aside, medical student, student physician and student doctor "can mean almost anything, and therefore mean very little. There is no clear role implied by the names students use at the time of introduction."[4] I use the term "medical student" in clinic for pragmatic reasons, namely, to use a term the patient will hopefully understand specifically in the context of my lack of licensure and curing capabilities. After establishing this basic element of honesty and trust, the most meaningful part of the entire process occurs when I begin to dialogue with the patient, at eye level, leaning slightly forward, completely focused on her illness narrative. The name I use is not important to me, but it might be important to the patient. Who patients perceives I am will affect how they allow me to accompany them. The experience of accompanying individuals is what I, and probably they, find to be most meaningful.

Questions

1. What *should* a medical student be called, and why?

2. How have you chosen to identify yourself to patients? Why? Has this changed during different points in your training? In what situations have you chosen one introduction over another? Does the name you use change the relationship between you and the patient?

3. Do you agree that the clinical encounter is a performance in which the medical student and patient are both actors and audience? To the extent this is true, what are the positive and negative implications of this performance?

4. Do you correct patients or their families if they are confused about your role on their care team? How do you do this, and what language do you use?

—Aleena Paul

On Empathy
(Can These Shoes Ever Fit?)

January 23, 2015

Jennifer Hong
Emory School of Medicine
Class of 2018

T HE POSITION OF AN M0.5 is a very paradoxical one. We've gone through five months of class, amazed that our brains can fit in so much material and even more amazed that we have to make room for more. We've gotten our white coats and try to ask patients smart questions while having no idea what solution we can provide for the ailments being enumerated. Our goal at this point is not to diagnose — it's to learn as much information as we can so that somewhere down the long, long line, we'll be able to utilize what we know and make something of it.

The majority of medical school so far has been learning about the science of living. It's the physiology, biochemistry, anatomy; the material that you pray that if you stare at the lectures long enough or watch enough Khan Academy videos, you'll eventually understand. And — fingers crossed — you probably will. The science is learnable because at the end of the day, it's the stuff you feel that you've just got to know, whether it's for the test in three weeks or for a diagnosis ten years down the line.

But in this age of patient-centered care, medical education cannot merely focus on the sciences. Knowing how to build rapport with patients is extremely important to a successful physician-patient relationship. Thus, another major component of this first year has been practicing how to talk with patients. In the past five months, I've thankfully practiced with standardized patients who've kindly understood why I've asked them three times in a row if they had a fever. When it comes to clinical applications, learning comes from the patient interactions themselves.

One of the most common feedbacks I've heard standardized patients give to first-years is something along the lines of, "I can really feel your empathy, that you care, and that's great." In the vein of learning how to interact with patients, this concept of empathy is something that crops up often —

after all, a good doctor is an empathetic one. We are told that there are certain ways you can show empathy: a consoling hand on the shoulder, a softer tone of voice, steady eye contact, the occasional nod. All these convey one message: I understand and I care.

Yet, as much as I appreciate and strongly believe we do need the classes focusing on clinical skills, I can't help but wonder — exactly how effective are these classes? Sure, you can teach students how to appear empathetic, but can you ever teach *anyone* to actually empathize? Essentially, it's the question that doctors have asked for decades already — can we actually be taught to care?

In Margaret Edson's Pulitzer Prize-winning play "W;t," Professor Vivian Bearing is a college English professor diagnosed with stage IV ovarian cancer. She agrees to be part of a clinical study, where she meets Jason Posner, a clinical fellow who had taken her 17th-century poetry class during his undergraduate years. Jason is the archetypal research-oriented physician who cares too deeply about the science of the disease but lacks insight into how the science manifests in patients' lives. After one morning's grand rounds, where Jason expertly presents Vivian's case to the team, he is prepared to leave when his attending prompts, "Clinical." Reminded, Jason turns to Vivian and says, "Thank you, Professor Bearing. You've been very cooperative."

It's easy to distance ourselves from Jason, a character who seems offensively stereotypical as the socially clueless doctor who clearly still has not "mastered" the "bedside manner." When reading this line, I typically picture Jason saying this statement in a rehearsed, mechanical way. But "W;t" is a play, meant to be spoken aloud, and without any stage direction, Jason's phrase could manifest in multiple manners: perhaps mechanically, perhaps coldly, but also perhaps kindly, warmly, empathetically. If the latter were true, what would change if Jason *had* mastered the bedside manner — just its presentation, and not its entity?

Empathy is often likened to understanding. Unlike sympathy or pity, which imply a hierarchy ("I feel sad *for* you, let *me* help *you*."), empathy connotes feeling for someone else because we understand them. Empathy is the feeling that results from understanding that we *could* be them, and therefore we care. Supposedly by understanding the experiences of patients or anyone around us, we can empathize because we can imagine ourselves in their positions.

Yet, this logic is faulty. To assume that we *could be them*, that only by possibly being them can we understand why we should care is not only flawed, but also self-imposing and hugely self-important. It is the same logic employed by many to convince others why rape culture exists — "imagine if it were your mother, your sister, your daughter." By this argument, we care only when we imagine how rape culture directly impacts us or someone we love, not because it is fundamentally terrible and damaging to others and to society as a whole. In the context of medicine, this process defeats the purpose of patient-centered care. Not only does this place our personal feelings at the forefront, it also invalidates the actual patient experience.

Furthermore, to "walk in the shoes" of patients is a grand assumption. In "W;t," Jason assumes he understands Vivian as the strict, imposing professor he had and therefore assumes that he understands Vivian's condition. As such, he assumes that Vivian is capable of pushing forward with rounds of chemotherapy without difficulty. By holding her to a standard created from his own projection of understanding, he completely silences Vivian's pain and her wishes. This culminates at the end of the play in his attempt to forcibly resuscitate Vivian despite her DNR.

More damaging than lack of understanding is the invalidation of a patient or any marginalized individual's experience by assuming that we do understand. Can Jason, a healthy, young man truly imagine the experiences of a woman with stage IV ovarian cancer? Similarly, can I, a young, healthy student, truly "understand" the experiences of a patient three times my age? The answer is undoubtedly, "No." We cannot empathize with all our patients. I highly doubt we can actually empathize with any of our patients, unless we've been in the same exact conditions.

This leaves us with a conundrum: why teach clinical skills when we can't fully understand? Are these classes useless then?

Of course not. Clinical skills are crucial and important; being able to care for patients is both an innate characteristic and a skill that can be honed. But caring for a patient does not necessarily require understanding their experiences in the sense that we can imagine ourselves in them. Rather than learning these skills in the context of empathy, we should be learning them in the context of acknowledgment. Instead of caring for patients because we understand them, we should be caring for patients in spite of understanding them, for only then do we practice actual *patient*-centered care: care for the patient's emotions, experiences, and understanding, not our own.

Questions

1. Do you agree with the author's statement that "we cannot empathize with all of our patients"? Why or why not?

2. Is it possible to provide humanistic care for patients *without* being empathetic?

3. Is it possible to teach empathy? Are clinical skills classes a vital part of medical education, or are they condescending?

4. The author argues that teaching empathy is self-centered rather than patient-centered, using the example of Jason in "W;t." Do you agree or disagree, and why?

—Aleena Paul

Learning to See: On Photography, Narrative, and Medical Education
February 5, 2015

Olivia Low
Albert Einstein College of Medicine
Class of 2018

PHOTOGRAPHY TAUGHT ME how to see. It taught me to listen using my eyes, rather than my ears alone.

This is something that I have carried with me throughout the beginning of medical school. Though some people assume that the arts and the sciences do not mix, photography has actually informed how I envision my work as a physician. In fact, I believe that many forms of creative practice have the ability to teach us lessons relevant to patient care.

Before I moved from California to New York to start college, my dad gave his old Nikon to me. It was clunky, and I did not know how to use it. But it felt right to hold it in my hands. As I awoke to the visual world around me, the way that I saw it physically changed. I began to look for details and make observations as I walked around the streets of New York. It was as if I had put on glasses for the first time, and everything had suddenly come into focus. I would find birdhouses in the hidden gardens of the East Village, dramatic geometries of the city's skyscrapers, and new shades of blue in the berries at the farmer's market. The way that the sunset would softly touch someone's hair reminded me of the everyday beauty that exists. The delicate intricacies of everyday life became more apparent, and thus, more significant.

One warm spring day, I went to the botanical garden with one of my friends. Trees with luscious, pale pink petals, grassy fields and flowers of all colors enveloped us. Though my friend had faced her share of hardships recently, I sensed a change in her that day. She was climbing trees and hiking through the forest in a way that made it seem like she was shedding a layer of misery and reemerging as a new soul. She felt free.

Because I had my camera with me, I wanted to capture this moment. When looking through the viewfinder, I began to pay attention. Where did her gaze fall? What was she doing with her hands? How did she fit into her environment? The process of photographing her became a dance between us in which we each reacted to one another. With every photo I took, I sought to elicit and interpret her personal story.

Making a portrait of someone is an intimate experience, much like a conversation with a patient. In both cases, I want the person I am with to feel cared for, valued and comfortable. Both require a certain kind of respect, earned trust and a willingness to sit back and watch.

When we gather a patient's history, we use all of our senses, including sight. Visual clues that patients give, such as their body language or facial expressions, lead to important diagnoses and better understandings of their emotions. Perceiving these subtleties allows us to respond with greater empathy and sensitivity, which likely results in better care. Now, when I encounter patients, I do my best to listen with my eyes.

Photographing people taught me that the active search for someone's narrative is essential to human connection. That connection is sacred and lies at the heart of medicine.

Given how much photography has enriched my appreciation for the humanity of others, I wish to encourage medical students to also nourish the creative parts of themselves. This is not about the result, but rather the practice itself. Things as simple as keeping a journal, buying a watercolor set, or reading books from diverse authors can help us expand our capacity for imagination. Activities like these do not need to be seen as outside of medical school, but rather integrated into our process of learning and growth.

As medical students, we are warned that our empathy will fade with time and that our emotional intelligence will falter. We need to address this problem with broad changes to our education, and it is worth considering a wide array of solutions that we can try now to stem this tide.

Medical schools seek to develop "humanistic" physicians, but what does that really mean? Perhaps that means incorporating things that both encourage us to reflect on our own transformation and push us to deepen our consciousness of others. If that is the case, the arts and humanities have the potential to play a meaningful role in this journey.

Questions

1. Do you have any hobbies or passions unrelated to medicine that shape how you approach medical school or how you view your patients? How so?

2. Do you use art, music, literature, film, or dance as an escape from medicine, or do you incorporate your medical life into your art?

3. How often do you "listen with your eyes" when seeing a patient? What details have you been able to pick up from body language, facial expressions, and other unspoken forms of communication?

4. Do you think the arts and humanities should be incorporated into medical education? Why or why not? Should those courses be required, or elective? Why or why not?

—Nisha Hariharan

30 Percent Bucket

February 23, 2015

Joshua Stein
Columbia University College of Physicians and Surgeons
Class of 2018

"CHUVASH POLYCYTHEMIA," Sue declares. "That's going in my 30 percent bucket."

We are studying for our upcoming molecular mechanisms test, as part of the semester-long course intended to introduce us to the basic functions of molecules, cells and tissues. In this integrated curriculum, all the names have changed, and the organization of the material is promised to magically improve our comprehension and recollection of such details.

However, Sue and I have a sneaking suspicion that we are actually taking pathology! We are lectured at by *pathologists*, we have daily *pathology* lab and we are using a classic *pathology* textbook. I have yet to taste any samples, but if I did, I am sure they would taste like pathology.

"How full is your bucket?" I inquire. Sue clasps her fingers in the air, around an imaginary handle. She carefully weighs it.

"Feels like I'm at around 20 percent."

"Excellent. Keep it in the bucket. Unless you are planning a trip to Chuvashia..."

As first-year medical students, we are undertaking a rite of passage, which we will one day fondly recall to our grandchildren. We are flooded with information — more than can be humanly absorbed — and then left to pick out what we think is important. On our exams, which are pass-fail, we are required to answer 70 percent of the questions correctly. Hence the imaginary bucket, into which we can safely discard up to 30 percent of everything we are taught.

While the selection process could be random (we could simply study material taught on Monday through Thursday and "bucket" Friday's lecture), most students guide their selection by what it deemed to be "high yield." Through an ever-evolving game of telephone, older students relay what is important to each individual professor.

As it turns out, Sue has to "unbucket" chuvash polycythemia, because professor B *always* asks a question about it. The man has an abiding concern for the Chuvashians. Yet no matter the process, we all live in fear of dumping out our buckets later, and finding something vital that we missed in the torrent.

As much as we are enjoying this ritual of the preclinical years, there is an equally satisfying, and even more ubiquitous tradition waiting for us on the other side of the USMLE Step 1: forgetting it all. In an informal, non-scientific survey conducted by the author this afternoon, 0 percent (+/- the hematologists) of hospital attendings can recall the molecular details of the coagulation cascade (n=10, including a few relatives). The following are a sample of responses:

> "I do remember that it exists, and is important so that one doesn't bleed to death!" —anonymous attending, fellowship director with over 25 years in practice

> "Nope. Of course, I didn't do so well on this exam in medical school..." —anonymous department chair

> "Wikipedia, dude." —medical resident in need of a shower and shave

In summary, first- and second-year medical students are flooded with information that may or may not be important (see "chuvash polycythemia"), of which they learn approximately 70 percent, half of which they promptly forget, and replace with clinically relevant knowledge, such as how to access UpToDate.

The question we must ask ourselves is simple: is this the best way to educate doctors?

As a medical community, we should demand more than 70 percent acquisition of information that we believe could one day be lifesaving to our patients. Nobody wants a nuclear inspector who is 70 percent protecting us from disaster. Nobody wants to be taken care of by an intern that scraped by with a barely passing grade. As students, we cannot be reasonably expected to learn more, learn thoroughly, and retain it all. The solution, unfortunately, requires more than clever teaching devices like "flipped lessons" or an integrated curriculum (both excellent ideas, but not sufficient). Perhaps it is time to fundamentally refocus the medical school curriculum on the clinically relevant, reduce the amount of *required* information, and raise our standards for what constitutes mastery of the basics.

Questions

1. As a medical student facing overwhelming amounts of information to learn, how do you make the decision about which information is necessary and which is expendable?

2. Do you believe that the ability to remember esoteric information correlates to your capability as a future physician? Why or why not?

3. This article calls for educational reform. If you could, what would you change about your preclinical years to make your classroom time more valuable?

—Nisha Hariharan

On Clinical Teaching and Evidence-Based Medicine

March 4, 2015

Amy Briggs
Keck School of Medicine of the University of Southern California
Class of 2016

E VIDENCE-BASED MEDICINE is a topic about which we as medical students hear lectures, have workshops and complete written assignments. What is it really? Is it just keeping up with the most recent literature in the field of medicine and practicing medicine based on evidence? The reason I bring up these questions is because I recently scrubbed in on a surgery during which I was not entirely sure if I was witnessing evidence-based medicine in practice, and this made me feel distinctly uncomfortable.

I had been invited by an attending to scrub in on a hysterectomy, which I appreciated as the clinical site I had been assigned to provided somewhat limited gynecologic surgery exposure. I had not been working on this attending's service, so I did not know anything about the patient, and had never met her. As we walked, I asked the attending more about the case. What was the indication for the hysterectomy? Bleeding, caused by a large fibroid. How old was the patient? 50. Would this hysterectomy be open or laparoscopic? His response to my last question was something like this: "I am not trained in laparoscopy, and besides, this is not the university hospital. Everyone there is on salary but working here, I am running a business. I do not have five hours to spend doing a hysterectomy." This response was, I think understandably, a little off-putting. The principles my attending seemed to be using to make this decision did not appear to be the right ones. I wondered if he was making a sound business decision rather than what might have been a better clinical decision.

Let's give my attending the benefit of the doubt. He is not trained in laparoscopy and it would be unsafe for him to attempt a laparoscopic surgery. Although there are good data that show that laparoscopic hysterectomy relative to abdominal hysterectomy is associated with shorter hospital stays, fewer wound infections, less blood loss and a faster return to normal activity, it is by no means the standard of care. We did not even discuss vaginal hysterectomy as an option even though there are benefits to this approach as well. It is likely that my attending considered that route but decided the fibroid was too large (and it was quite large) and that an abdominal hysterectomy was the best, safest surgery he could provide. Perhaps he also considered that continuity of care is valuable to both patients and providers, and that was why he chose not to refer her to someone who does laparoscopy. Additionally, one could make the argument that physicians have a duty to provide care to as many patients as they are able and if doing abdominal hysterectomies allows a physician to maximize the number of patients he is able to treat, then he should do so. These were the rationalizations that I came up with in the absence of a more thorough explanation from my attending.

We completed the surgery with the assistance from a second attending and as we were leaving, I asked my attending why he had made the decision to remove the ovaries. I vaguely remembered hearing from a resident that the ovaries continue to produce hormones for ten to 15 years after menopause and that removing them at the time of hysterectomy was no longer routine. His response was along the lines of "they have the potential to get cancer and she's 50, so they're not doing much anyway." By his tone, I could tell he was not especially interested in discussing the case any further. I read about oophorectomies when I went home that night. I learned that there are several indications for an oophorectomy in a fifty-year-old woman at the time of hysterectomy, including the reason my attending had cited. However, the benefits of oophorectomy in these women, especially women without known ovarian pathology or family history of ovarian cancer, must be weighed against the risks. These risks include an increase in all-cause mortality, cardiovascular disease and neurologic disease. The degree of risk is dependent on the age of the patient at oophorectomy and whether or not the patient takes supplemental estrogen after the procedure. I chose to believe that my attending was well aware of all of this evidence and that he had had a lengthy discussion with the patient about the risks and benefits of oophorectomy prior to the surgery.

In this situation, what is my ethical responsibility? Much of the onus lies on us as medical students to educate ourselves about our patients and the therapies we provide. We need to know the evidence. If I had known more about the procedure my patient was undergoing, I could have asked better questions, questions like, "Did you and the patient decide on what you were going to do regarding estrogen supplementation after the surgery?" or "Does the patient have any risk factors for cardiovascular disease?" Some of the responsibility also lies with our residents and attendings to help us understand why they make the clinical decisions they make and how they integrate the evidence into their own practice. The patient demographics and individual patient preferences that a clinician encounters may influence his or her recommendations in ways that are not necessarily readily apparent to an observer. It is the harmony of evidence, the patient's needs and a clinician's judgment that truly makes medicine both a science and an art.

Questions

1. Define "evidence-based medicine" in terms of what it means to you. How will you incorporate it in your medical practice?

2. Have you ever participated in or witnessed care that was less than evidence-based? How did you react?

3. Can you think of any scenarios in which evidence-based medicine could act as a barrier to care?

4. Do you agree with the author's recommendation to harmonize evidence-based medicine with patient needs and clinical judgment? What have you seen in practice?

5. What strategies can help ensure that we effectively utilize an evidence-based approach to patient care?

—Nikki Nametz Feinberg

The Value of Empathy in Medicine

March 6, 2015

Sarah Bommarito
Wayne State University School of Medicine
Class of 2016

EMPATHY: IT'S WHAT supposedly drives us to become physicians, and what we're told to demonstrate through our extracurricular activities and during our interviews. We yearn for that perfect patient interaction in which we comforted or understood in a way that changed the patient's perspective on medical care. In our idealized view of medicine, we truly believe that empathy will be our saving grace throughout medical school, residency and beyond. If we can simply connect with our patients, then we will succeed and the patients we care for will thrive.

And then we begin our clinical rotations.

During orientation at my clinical site, one of the attending physicians gave a presentation on how to avoid becoming "robots" during the course of our medical training. I sat in the audience and wondered how I could ever fully disregard emotion, but the entire premise of the speaker's presentation hinged on the certainty that this would happen unless we tried very, very hard to remain human. I considered this for a while and decided that while I could understand how some of my classmates might lose empathy, my hyper-empathic tendencies simply could never be diminished. After all, studies have shown that physician burnout is worsened by forcing down negative feelings that naturally occur over years of bending to the burden of patient care.

In the following days and weeks I kept this lecture in the back of my mind as I began to learn how to interact with difficult patients, take overly detailed histories, complete monotonously thorough physical exams, and present this information to my often-impatient superiors. Early on I realized that when you're part of a medical team, empathy isn't valued nearly as highly as virtues such as efficiency, confidence and medical knowledge — and did I mention efficiency?

Many aspects of clinical care can be reduced to measures of time. Insurance companies become vocal if they have to pay for a longer length of stay. Patients become irritable if you ask seemingly similar questions too many times — even though we've all seen that slight rewordings of a question can yield strikingly different answers during rounds. The interns to whom you're assigned are too swamped with paperwork to care about the fact that your patient is apprehensive about being discharged and wants more information before leaving. The attending physician has to be somewhere this afternoon, and how could you even consider bringing up patients' trivial concerns when there are lab values to be discussed and additional tests to be ordered before lunch?

It isn't that one part of the system demands efficiency — it's that most parts do. In order to function as a valuable member of a medical team, you almost have to conform to these standards. People and companies expect this from you. You learn to optimize the amount of work you can do and the number of patients you can see in a morning and an afternoon, and the standards continue to become more rigorous.

During my second rotation, I was placed on an oncology floor. In the beginning, I often inconspicuously shared in the sense of sadness and hopelessness that my patients and their families faced when trying to understand their diagnoses and prognoses. I learned not to go to my superiors with details of personal talks with patients after being told and reminded that I wasn't allowed to be sad after long discussions about impending death. It was my job to be strong for patients so they wouldn't see tears in my eyes and assume that all hope was lost.

Within a few short weeks, I had accepted that stage IV cancer could be equated to certain death in a shorter amount of time than any patient was ready to accept, and I had even begun to think somewhat negatively of patients and family members who stubbornly refused to agree with these now-obvious realities. In large part, this way of thinking shielded me from the pain of relating to these patients. I began to think that medical professionals might be on to something: maybe it's right to disregard empathy in favor of a more logical approach to patients, a bedside manner that is more realistic than overtly comforting.

However, I was forced to reconsider this idea. This way of thinking caused me more exhaustion and misery than I had ever felt in my medical training. I went home with headaches, complained about my day and then holed up to study. While I enjoyed learning about medical conditions, I felt little emotional pull to continue my day-to-day work.

And then a patient and his family put me back on track. The patient, middle-aged and in a relatively new marriage, had been diagnosed with stage IV cancer about two weeks before I first met him. When we first spoke, he was irritable and quick to disregard me. His wife apologized for him several times during the difficult interview. I told her I understood that he was in a great deal of pain and exhaustion and appreciated their patience with me.

Over the next few days, she began to tell me details of her husband's illness that never came up during rounds.

The patient declined slowly at first and then, after a routine procedure, his mental status became severely altered. No available treatment could prevent further decline. The team recommended hospice care to keep him comfortable. His wife, though upset, seemed to understand, but admitted that she needed time to think and to discuss this with their immediate family.

By the time I went to the patient's room to check on him later in the day, his wife's attitude had changed drastically. She began to accuse the team of giving up on her husband. She told me that he was a good man who had provided for his kids for many years. He was a hard worker. He cared so much about her. Why did he get worse so suddenly? She wasn't ready to give up on him; why was our team giving up?

I listened to her with conflicting emotions. I knew this was difficult for her, but I also knew from my admittedly small amount of experience that the best thing to do was to ensure his comfort in his final days. But something in this woman's tone sank into me and reminded me that we were dealing with a unique patient. She hadn't faced this situation before. This is easy to forget after seeing so many patients with similar afflictions. Even in the small amount of time I had been on the service, I began to comprehend that physicians become used to certain situations despite changing patients. Disregarding a patient's individuality allows for treating the condition based on medically sound evidence without the need to understand the patient's whole story. This certainly saves time and energy that may be better spent on other tasks, after all.

At the end of the woman's tangential musings she began to cry — quietly at first, and then with sobs that shook her body. Without considering my actions, I moved a box of tissues closer to her and placed my hand on her shoulder. I told her that we weren't giving up on her husband, and that we would do everything in our power to decrease his pain and maintain his comfort. I told her I knew her husband was a good man just by seeing how much she and their family cared for him, and that the team would be there to answer her questions and do as much as possible for her and her husband. My sentiments were genuine. Nothing I could have said would have soothed her entirely, but she was noticeably less upset and more open to considering the difficult decision at hand.

Empathy didn't save the patient's life, of course. He passed away comfortably under hospice care a couple of weeks later. But that day — in that moment — I knew I had improved the situation simply by seeing the patient's humanity and relating to his wife. While our conversation did not make the decision for her, it seemed to give her a sense of peace in making a difficult decision. Because of her decision, her husband was ultimately granted comfort in his final moments.

A later experience during my psychiatry clerkship provided further support for the value of empathy. I was placed at an addiction treatment facility for two weeks and primarily saw outpatient encounters. One day, I was invited to a group therapy session in which the patients wrote letters to their addictions and the residents and students wrote letters to those suffering from addiction. I wrote about how I hoped patients would find support, care, comfort and acceptance in us and how proud we are that they were taking the necessary steps to find clarity and overcome their addictions to lead healthier, more fulfilling lives. In short, I told them we're on their side.

While I wasn't able to stay to hear many of the letters, the therapist later told me that when she read our letters to the group, the patients became very emotional. They hadn't realized how much we cared, she said, and it changed their perspectives on seeking care from physicians after their stay at the facility. Many of them had felt discouraged at their appointments and assumed that we saw them as a nuisance. In reality, many of us saw them as strong and determined people who were ready to get back on track and repair their damaged relationships and lives through treatment.

Showing empathy to patients can mean more than we realize or understand. Simply knowing that someone truly cares can help patients feel comfortable and justified in seeking the appropriate treatment or making a difficult medical decision.

As medical students, we're in the unique situation of experiencing some amount of responsibility to care for patients as well as the time to do so in a way that many residents and attending physicians cannot. Our time isn't billed to insurance companies, and there are so many options when it comes to how we can choose to spend it. I realize that I will reach a point where my time will become more limited, when I might find myself in a more robotic state with the eightieth patient who presents with a certain condition, but I hope I find the strength to return to this empathic state of mind at least as often as I leave it. I hope no one is ever able to fully convince me that empathy in medicine isn't worth the effort.

In continued lectures, I am reminded that empathic interactions need not take more than a couple minutes to make a positive impact, and I've seen that a couple minutes is often enough to show a patient that you truly care about his or her outcome and that you are undoubtedly on his or her side. Sometimes patients and their families need to feel that sense of shared concern in order to feel comforted and adequately cared for. Sometimes physicians need to remember that their patients are human in order to avoid a sense of emptiness in their careers.

I am often given cause to wonder, even if the interaction takes slightly longer, what do we have to lose by showing concern, listening to our patients, and allowing ourselves to hold on to that feeling that drove us to become physicians in the first place? In truth, it seems that, to the contrary, we all have so much to gain.

Questions

1. What do you think is the link between empathy and burnout? Does empathy cause burnout or protect against it?

2. Do you think that diminished empathy is more common in some medical specialties than others? Which ones? Why do you think that is the case?

3. Have you ever had an experience in which you just couldn't connect with a patient? How did it make you feel? How do you think the patient felt?

4. Finding the right balance between treating the condition and treating the individual can be difficult at times. What strategies can you think of to effectively address both the disease and the person at one time?

5. Some people deal with difficult diagnoses through the coping mechanism of "intellectualization" in which they choose to deal only with the facts of their condition rather than the emotional impact. How can you use empathy effectively with these patients?

—Lindsey McDaniel

"May I Ask You a Few Questions and Examine You?"

March 30, 2015

Tania Tabassum
Dubai Medical College
Class of 2015

D URING OUR MEDICAL TRAINING, taking a proper history and doing a thorough clinical examination within a limited time period are the two skills that we are expected to master perfectly. Our teachers tell us that a good history gives you 75 percent of your diagnosis and the clinical examination gets you 90 to 100 percent of the diagnosis.

But what is a good history? A good history consists of all the positive findings, the important negative findings, family history, social history, marital history. And the fact that you need to obtain all this information means that you can't be talking about things that have nothing to do with the patients' medical condition. You can't be spending five minutes discussing the game last week or what the patient's son has been up to lately. We are supposed to stop our patients and direct them back to the problem at hand. We expect a person to disclose all their details to us — what they ate last night, how many times they went to the bathroom, when was the last time they had sexual intercourse, if they smoke or drink, who they live with — after we tell them nothing about ourselves except our name and designation.

A very widely accepted statement when beginning an OSCE (objective structured clinical exam) station is: "Hello Mr./Miss (insert name), I am (insert name), I am a medical student. I would like to ask you a few questions so that we can have a better understanding of what's going on with you in order to help you. Is that okay?"

We begin by saying that we are here to help them and we always expect them to answer in the affirmative. What do they have to complain about? After all, we are here to serve their purpose: antibiotics for the infection and analgesics for the pain. So we feel entitled to it. But have you ever considered exactly how much we are asking of them?

It is normal for us, medical professionals, to ask these personal questions on a regular basis. But for the patient, we are strangers. They are not used to discussing their life stories with everyone and yet, we think it's unreasonable if they refuse to disclose a detail. We fail to understand why it might be awkward for a person to talk about how stressful their work is or how their living conditions are, when they only came to the emergency room for an episode of loss of consciousness. More often than not, patients have to disclose this information in front of a room full of people: the medical student taking the history, the second student who is taking notes, the nurse who is putting on a dressing, the phlebotomist who is drawing blood for labs. Later, we return with the doctor, two interns and three other students, and present our case. The patient lies quietly in bed while we disclose their entire life — the fall they had as a child, the bottle of wine they finished the night before, where they work and where they live — to a room full of strangers. And while we do this to people on a daily basis, how willing are we to have the same thing done to us?

A few weeks ago, during one of the teaching sessions, the doctor wanted to demonstrate how to do a diabetic foot examination. One of my friends volunteered to be the surrogate patient. The doctor first did a general examination and then proceeded to do the foot examination while we all crowded around the bed to watch. She later told me that it was one of the most embarrassing moments of her life. Why? Because there were 10 different people watching while she was being examined; her feet and legs were exposed to the knee; she felt awfully self-conscious to be lying like that in front of so many people and have a person describe her feet in great details to an audience. Yet, we complain about those patients who refuse to let us do a physical on them, the patients who refuse to let us expose them in front of a total stranger, and be touched and poked and auscultated. After all, if we don't practice and we don't learn, who is going to treat them? But then why is it that when we are the ones being put in the same position for the sake of education, we complain?

There is no denying that this is the only way to learn. The more we practice, the better physicians we will become. But we must remember what we take from our patients during the process of learning. Because no, we are not entitled to the details they give us. We are privileged. No, the patients aren't just supposed to let us invade their personal space. We are supposed to apologize for exposing them and explain why it is absolutely necessary. It isn't just us who are doing them a massive favor by diagnosing and treating them; they are doing us a favor by letting us practice on them and learn.

It is very easy to forget during the long years of training and later during our years of practice that there isn't much of a difference between ourselves and the people we treat. The people we socialize with outside the hospital are the same people we encounter in the hospital. They deserve to be treated with the same amount of respect. Our patients aren't diagnoses or a bunch of interesting clinical findings. They are people who deserve to be thanked for allowing us to examine them, apologized to for the discomfort we are causing them, and empathized with when they refuse to allow us to do so. Always stop to think: if you were the person lying in a hospital bed in pain, instead of being the person doing the questioning, how would you like to be treated?

Questions

1. Have you ever served as a standardized patient to help your classmates learn an aspect of the physical exam? How did that make you feel?

2. Put yourself in the place of a patient in a teaching hospital: a student comes in to question and examine you before the sun has come up, and then a bit later a resident does a slight variation of the same thing. Then, hours later a team of strangers walks into your room: the attending, the resident and student assigned to your case, and likely a few more residents and students, and possibly nurses, pharmacists, or therapists as well. They ask personal questions and expect answers. If you have a unique exam finding, you may find yourself being asked to allow three or four people you don't know to examine you briefly. How do you react? How does this make you feel? Should patients at a teaching hospital expect to be interviewed and examined by all kinds of learners?

3. The author of this piece calls it a privilege to be able learn from patients in ways that often compromise their privacy. Do you agree that this is a privilege? As a student of medicine, what other privileges do you have?

4. How can you as a student improve the privacy and comfort of patients without sacrificing the quality of your education?

—Lindsey McDaniel

Overthink It!

April 13, 2015

Eric Donahue
University of Washington School of Medicine
Class of 2017

M Y CLASSMATES AND PROFESSORS tell me I overthink it. "You over-analyzed the problem." "Stop mulling it over." "Just focus on the buzz-words and you'll rock the exam." "Jump through the hoops and move on."

But I cannot. I refuse to give into the bureaucracy! The qualities of my character — namely an unrelenting stubbornness — drive me to full-on dis-sidence against the cliché "don't overthink it." The phrase makes my skin crawl. It insults my intelligence by undermining the very passions that drew me to medicine in the first place.

I did not pursue this long and arduous path because I desired wealth or admiration. Nor did I choose to achieve a career that was predictable or sim-ple. I sought the challenge of the unknown, to battle against time and death to solve the mysteries of the human condition. To provide hope and maybe a few second chances to those in pain and desperation. I wanted a career where at the end of the day, no matter what the outcome, I knew I gave my all to those I was responsible for.

After almost two years in medical school I have become eerily aware that we are being prepared for "conveyor belt medicine." A fictional world where patients present with well-explained, easily treatable problems that require nothing more than an algorithm and a 25 percent probability of guessing the right answer. A place where zebras are more commonplace than cats and every patient is compliant and trustworthy.

Just imagine it: Mr. Smith strolls into your office and gives you a 10 sec-ond synopsis of his symptoms — revealing a few juicy buzzwords in the process. Then he removes his gown and you follow the instructions pinned to his chest:

For strep throat, circle the mouth. For coronary artery disease, circle the left nipple. For gastroenteritis, circle the navel. And for sexually transmitted infections ... you get the idea.

You mark your answer, then send the patient on his way down the conveyor belt. In his hand, a prescription, a satisfaction survey and a cherry lollipop to seal the deal. All in a day's work — nailed it!

The truth is real life patients rarely present the way they do on multiple-choice exams. The answers to their problems are seldom solved by one or two novel treatments. They have genetic, social, religious and even spiritual facets that contribute to the complexity of their condition. Many times, the unknown persists and as their providers we will be forced to accept this. However, appreciating that some problems cannot be solved is not an excuse for complacency. We are called to exhaust our minds and to employ our passion for the benefit of our patients.

Sir Arthur Conan Doyle was a writer and a physician in the late 1800s. His character Sherlock Holmes has become a staple in my digestion of literature over the years. Holmes solved every crime with such eccentric enthusiasm, devoting the depths of his brilliance to each case and was astutely observant to every detail. In the mind of this genius, nothing occurred by happenstance. Everything had a purpose and a contribution. His neurotic passion was infectious. I thought to myself, "If I could contain even a fraction of this character's brilliance, oh the mysteries I would solve!"

It was not until recently I learned that the character Sherlock Holmes was actually inspired by a physician, Joseph Bell. Rumor states that he was very much like the man in those famed stories. However instead of solving crime, he solved disease. I like to imagine that he did so with every bit of passion and tenacity as the character he inspired. He was an overthinker. A true physician.

The next time a professor tells you that you're overthinking it, just bite your tongue and jump through their hoop. But agree to disagree and never stop overthinking it. You may not receive admiration from the academic world and you may not receive the high score on the test. But be true to yourself and your patients will benefit from that commitment. That, my friends, is what matters most.

Questions

1. Does performance on medical school exams or standardized board exams reflect one's aptitude to be a good physician? What other qualities are necessary?

2. What are some of the cognitive traps to avoid so that patient interviews do not become *pro forma*, as the author suggests?

3. You will spend years learning and taking exams, and you will become a proficient test-taker. How do you transition your ability to convey knowledge on a multiple-choice exam to actual patient care and clinical reasoning? Are there ways to foster this transition early in your training?

4. As you progress through your training, how will you retain the passion that drew you to medicine in the first place? How will you take ownership of your learning, not just to perform well academically, but more importantly to use that knowledge for your future patients?

—Eric Donahue

Work-Life Balance

Eau de Medical School

March 13, 2014

Nita Chen
Albany Medical College
Class of 2017

At the start, it was
Crisp
Like the sound of a chilled cucumber
Snapped in half briskly on a hot summer day
Fresh
In the novelty of all things
A foreign state with foreign friends
A foreign box to call a home.
With time, it was replaced with
The reek
Of persistent formaldehyde
Clinging to every pore
And every item owned
(despite relentless efforts to sterilize and compartmentalize)
Its phantom stench in almost every aroma perceived
(whether imagined or real)
Like
The way medical school had become a way of life
Instead of
Just one of the things we do.
And as the formaldehyde settled in
Noses learned to readjust to its background presence
Minds became accustomed to chronic weariness
And dopamine pathways permanently hooked onto
The pleasures of tea addictions.
(or simply caffeine, caffeine, caffeine — to each his own)
The appreciation of the small reliefs in life became essential

(treasure, oh, treasure the small things in life)
Like the comforting aroma of milk and Earl Grey
Or the dusty familiarity of Things From Home
Or even that aseptic cleanse of the winter snow.
But mostly, it is that fuzzy
Perfectly humidified air
Mixed in with the embers of last night's drying tea leaves
Where the most comfort is found as
The rest of the senses succumb in a cradle of
(smooth, rhythmically rocking)
beta and theta waves.

Questions

1. In this poem, the author uses vivid imagery and all five senses to demonstrate the all-encompassing feeling of medical school. Is medical education designed as an immersive experience, or does it simply become one because of the intensive nature of the training?

2. Do you feel like this immersion is valuable, or dangerous, and why?

3. Is it okay for medical school to become a "way of life"? Should there be a balance between personal identity and professional identity, and if so, how can medical students achieve this balance? How do you balance your personal life and professional life?

—Brent Schnipke

Doctor Dad: A Husband and Father of Three in Med School

April 10, 2014

Daniel Gates
Indiana University School of Medicine
Class of 2017

H OW DO YOU FIND a balance in medical school?
"There is no balance," she said.

This was not what I wanted to hear. We were talking about remaining competitive in medical school without giving up a social life. This administrator is an MD and has a PhD in education; she knows what she's saying. She explained how her eight-year-old gets a few hours after work, but then she often sacrifices sleep to stay on top of her professional to-do list.

I completely understand the demands of children. All three of mine expect their own bit of my attention, as well as participation in family time. Needless to say, the administrator was flabbergasted when I told her about my teenager, school-ager and toddler. This is not typical and the demand is immense but, with the right attitude and some perseverance, it is more than manageable. Three basic tenets guide me to successfully passing my classes without ignoring my children and abandoning their care to my wife.

After years of perfection, the 4.3 in high school and the 3.9 in undergrad, most medical students have spent years blowing the curve and displaying perfection in their work. This is the life we lead to make it to medical school. The Type A, perfection-seeking behavior is what makes us suitable to guard the health and safety of our patients. However, the old joke is not quite a joke after all; what do you call a med student that finishes at the bottom of his class? Doctor.

Many medical schools have a pass/fail grading system, with cutoffs for a passing grade as low as 60 percent. The average passing cutoff is in the range of 70 percent, which is a C in most places. I tell myself every day that the best thing I can do for my family at this point is to pass medical school, but the husband and father in me demand I do more than study all day and night. So, my first tenet is to give up on perfection. I'm speaking of academic perfection, since this is an absolutely arbitrary concept. I don't think merely passing my classes is acceptable, but I'm not a gunner, and I don't kill myself over getting a 77 percent on an exam.

Of course, I want to do more than simply pass my classes. I want to learn something that will one day save or improve the quality of life for one of my patients; this takes a new level of time management. While timing was never one of my strong suits (after all, who would choose to have three children, each five years apart), time management has been a major key to my success. Each week I have 168 hours with which to do all that I need to take care of my family and pass my classes. With about 50 of those taken up by sleep, 14 for eating, and about 30 dedicated to my family, I don't have much time for studying; using that time to its utmost is necessity.

At home, with your computer, and your TV, and your Playstation, and your friends, and ... you get the picture. Removing distractions is a difficult task, but removing yourself from those distractions is easy. Attending lectures, instead of viewing them online at home, is a prime way to aid focus. If you're like me, and you don't live near campus, going to the local library on the weekends is always an option. To distill this point, treat school like a job. Use the time you're on campus (you will actually need to go to campus) more effectively. Between classes, you should review material for the next class, or prepare questions about the class that just ended. Use lunch to read material or complete lab work (unless it's anatomy lab, as I don't condone skipping meals). When you get home, put work aside for a few hours to refresh yourself, and enjoy the time that you have with your family, because you can't get these days back, and they'll pass you by in a blink.

Finally, don't overdo it. Get enough sleep, and make sure you're eating healthily. In the long run, nutrition and sleep will go a long way. I spend about four hours every weeknight with my family: one hour cooking with my wife, one hour eating and asking my kids about their days, and two hours playing games with my daughters. Lunch is always packed the night before, as I'm the only one who will eat leftovers, and breakfast is an egg on toast, two oranges and some coffee. The kids all go to bed between 7 p.m. and 9 p.m., so I spend about two more hours reading the text or reviewing information for tomorrow's lectures; I wake up promptly at 6:30 a.m. to get ready for the day and to take my son to daycare on the way in to school. Only on very rare occasions do I feel that I didn't get enough sleep. I'm constantly hearing about fellow students staying up late to study, but then sleeping in and missing lecture. This kind of circadian disruption cannot last for long. Also, I hear about them eating out all the time because it's quick, or eating Chef Boyardee because it's cheap. Their breakfast usually consists of coffee and a candy bar. They aren't displaying any outward unhealthiness due to poor diet, but it must be there. We learn about the importance of proper diet and sleep, and we joke about not getting proper nutrition and sleep. I guess this is irony, or hypocrisy.

The average medical student is 23.5 years old; they are young and resilient and can stand to stay up late, miss lectures, eat poorly and they don't generally have dependents. However, I'm not so young anymore and family is the most important thing in the world to me. Perfection to me is a balanced home-work life. Medical school is not the typical 8 to 5 p.m. job, but neither is medicine in general. Yet it is still a job that we all hope to enjoy doing.

So I refuse to make it stressful and all-consuming. My time is valuable and so is my health. I'm a firm believer in practicing what I preach. I used to smoke (emphasis on "used to"). I can tell patients I know just how hard it is to quit, and how absolutely possible it is. I try to run, and walk if I can't run, at least every other day. I eat three meals a day and I sleep at least six hours a night. There is a balance. I'm not topping the grade reports, and I won't make it into Alpha Omega Alpha, but everyone will call me doctor just the same.

Questions

1. How do you find balance between being a student and being a person in medical school?

2. How do you set realistic goals for yourself during medical training? What do you prioritize outside of the classroom, and what do you sacrifice?

3. In medical school, you will be told what success looks like from every point of view. Overachievers and "gunners" will surround you. How do you define "success" in medical school? What are your personal goals and how will you devote yourself to them without being overwhelmed by the goals of those around you?

—Eric Donahue

Better Mom, Better Doctor

October 30, 2014

Mariya Cherneykina
Temple University School of Medicine
Class of 2017

F EW JOYS IN MY LIFE compare to that moment in November of 2011 when I opened that fateful letter granting me a spot in medical school. As I hopped for joy, I had no idea that I was celebrating with the person who would provide me with immeasurable joy for the rest of my life — the kind of joy that does not lend itself to metaphor, literary nuance or even the best descriptive talents.

A few short weeks later, he became real and tangible. First, he was a little mass that I could not touch, but could feel growing within me. Then, he grew to an audible inhabitant with the help of ultrasound. Finally, over weeks and months, he was a tumbling, hiccupping creature that seemed to live an independent life inside of me.

As acceptance deadlines approached, I was faced with my first conflict between being a mom and a future doctor. Anxiously, I contacted my school, nervous whether they would retract my admission, thinking that they would feel duped when I deliver a baby a mere two weeks into first year. The voice on the other line, however, was warm and understanding, reassuring me with complete support in whatever decision I would make. I was officially invited to the universal, yet somehow still exclusive, club called "motherhood." The decision was mine, the door was open, and my hard-earned spot would be there.

Much of that first year was spent with not enough sleep, covered in another human's bodily fluids, and feeling chronically stressed. However, the greater majority of it was the most rewarding, beautiful time of my life. Deferring medical school to stay home with my son for perhaps the most formative year of his life was the best decision for our family. I cherished our walks in the park, seeing him crawl around our living room, and even taking turns with my husband pacing with the baby in the middle of the night. Most importantly, because I knew this time was limited, I learned to imbibe every moment, to love and treasure in the present.

The first year of medical school was much like that first year. Yes, still sleep deprived, covered in foreign bodily fluids (though less cute than those that come from a baby), and still very much stressed. Add a mix of separation anxiety, trying to cook dinner with finals looming and a cranky toddler, and a sky-high pile of laundry, papers, books and projects. One could imagine that there was a solitary functioning neuron left in my brain, and it was tired. Many a night, my husband, my parents or my friends were consoling me from yet another mental ledge. I was constantly torn between wanting to be with my family and needing to study.

I was always asking why I was doing this to myself; I could have chosen a simpler career. After all, no one forced me to go to medical school. I could have stayed at home longer, given more of myself to my son and the rest of my family. Maybe I was not as strong as my mother, grandmother, great-grandmother and every female relative who had children while in medical school. However, at the end of the day, I knew that nothing could extinguish my desire to become a doctor. I knew that if I gave up, I would be a hypocrite telling my son to persevere when things got hard to achieve his dreams.

As I write this, now into my second year of medical school with my two-year-old comfortably sleeping next door, I am no longer teetering on that mental edge. I have since realized that who you are (mom, athlete, author) is never mutually exclusive with becoming a doctor. In fact, the more dimensions you can add to your medical career, the better you become. Being a mom made me more gentle, flexible and able to nurture in selfless ways I never understood before. Being a medical student makes me feel happy and fulfilled, something my child may only feel on some visceral level now, but will surely appreciate when he begins to pursue his own dreams. I still feel guilt pangs from time to time, but I just remind myself that becoming a better me, whether professionally or personally, will make me both a better doctor and a better mom.

Questions

1. Reflecting on this author's story, what challenges impacting work-life balance do you feel you will experience? Discuss how you and others can successfully navigate these challenges.

2. What is the importance of being both a person and a professional? How does your life outside of medicine make you a better physician? In what ways can the life outside medicine play a negative role?

3. Whether you have children now or plan to become a parent later in your training, how would this responsibility impact your approach to being a physician? How do you separate and fulfill responsibilities to your patients and to your children?

4. Do you think that, despite institutional rhetoric supporting work-life balance, medicine often asks you to prioritize work over home life? In that context, how would you pursue a balance?

—Eric Donahue

Never Forget Those Who Got You Here

February 22, 2015

Eric Donahue
University of Washington School of Medicine
Class of 2017

I N THE PURSUIT OF DREAMS, we are taught to never lose sight of our
goals. It is impossible to accomplish any meaningful ambition without a
devotion to discipline and the acceptance of personal sacrifice. This creates
tunnel vision, which is ideal for reaching a destination, but burdensome for
those close to you. It is easy to forget those who hold us up, push us forward
and who at the end of the day just say, "I love you, no matter what."

When I was 19 years old, I married the woman of my dreams. She was
beautiful! Perfect! Yet, in spite of this, I was still not satisfied with my life. She
stole my heart, but she could never tame my mind. It was rampant with pain
and confusion, tormented by the demands of finding purpose and meaning. Because of this I dragged her all over the world. Manila slums, island
jungles infested with insects, disease and even tribal war. Still, she never
complained. "I'm just happy to be with you, my love." Somewhere along the
way I decided my purpose was in medicine — to become a physician. I was
a 23-year-old high school dropout with absolutely no college or academic
success. Still, she never doubted me. "You can do it love, I know you can. I
believe in you."

She has always stayed by my side — almost 11 years now. She gave me
two beautiful daughters and right now she carries our son, all while glowing
like the stars. It has not always been easy. I worked full-time, went to college,
and did all those ridiculous things that we do to achieve our dream to be an
MD.

That did not leave a whole lot of time for her in my life. At times I imagine she felt abandoned, like a single mom. I'll admit it, I almost left more
than once. Almost gave up on all that love. Like many suited to pursue a
career in medicine, I am innately selfish, struggling with stubbornness and
insecurity. But she tells me, "your qualities are both a gift and a curse." I

am convinced that it is her life goal to bring out the good qualities in this grumpy soul.

The moral of the story is never to forget those who love you. They are your greatest gift in life, even if it is hard to see them in the tunnel of pursuit. They secretly give you the strength to become something special, something the world needs badly. Take a break from studying for the boards, take your furry friend for walk, call your mom, give your best friend a hug, and tell them what they mean to you. Give your significant other a kiss, a real one, and thank them. When you finish school, take them on a cruise. They deserve that and much, much more.

We may never be fully satisfied with our lives. We may never truly find peace of mind. But I think that's okay. This innate drive is what makes humanity great. It pushes us to discover, to cure disease, to stop hunger, and to make this place better. From the guy who will someday be a physician, here is a prescription that puts Valium to shame. Take 10 minutes out of your day, gaze on that beautiful one of yours and remember what made you fall in love them in the first place. Repeat as needed. (Don't worry, I can send unlimited refills to the pharmacy.)

Questions

1. Who are the people in your life who got you here? What words and sentiments would you like to convey to them?

2. Do you believe you have struggled with "stubbornness and insecurity" in your pursuit of medicine? If so, how has this affected your relationships outside of medicine?

—Aleena Paul

Being Pregnant During the First Year of Medical School

March 8, 2015

Allison Lyle
University of Louisville School of Medicine
Class of 2017

M Y STOMACH HAD BEEN in knots that morning.
"Are you pregnant?" my classmate laughed after I returned to the gross anatomy lab for the second time after leaving to get a drink.

"No," I chuckled, and returned to cutting through fat and fascia, teasing out the muscles and nerves for the day's dissection.

But, I wondered.

On the way home after lab, I bought a pregnancy test to put my mind at ease. Being in my late 20s when I began medical school, my husband and I had had many conversations about when would be an appropriate time to start a family during my training. The first sets of exams had gone well and I was getting plenty of time for myself while adjusting to life as a new medical student, so we had collectively thought I could handle being pregnant while in school. We had just begun trying to start a family, and I was convinced that there was no possible way I was already pregnant so soon.

However, the little "+" sign proved otherwise. We were both shocked and overwhelmingly excited to be parents. To be honest, though, I was also scared — now that I was actually pregnant, I wondered if my previous assessment of my abilities was overconfident. Was I so naïve that I thought I could be both a medical student and mother-to-be? Then, only a few months into my first year of medical school, I wondered if I could continue to be a good student while being pregnant.

Classes did nothing to ease my fears; at times, class content made my fears worse. When I first learned of the embryo I was carrying, my class was in the middle of medical embryology. As my pregnancy continued, those worries changed based on my newfound knowledge.

"You are not allowed to be a molar pregnancy," I would think toward my stowaway. "You are not allowed to have holoprosencephaly. You are not allowed to have a trisomy," I thought, as another wave of nausea would break my concentration.

Knowing that the majority of spontaneous abortions occur in the first eight weeks of development, I was not comfortable with sharing the news with anyone other than my husband — I was scared to death that I would miscarry. Sweatshirts and scrubs were my outfits of choice, my mechanism for concealing my secret until I was ready to share it. I was afraid that my professors and classmates would think that I was not a serious student since I had chosen to start a family during my training. (Luckily, my obstetrician was not on faculty, and was located near campus so I could easily attend my appointments without drawing suspicion.) Being a non-traditional student, I knew that my time frame for a family was different than some of my younger classmates', and I didn't want to be judged as incompetent because of my "condition."

As it happened, my "condition" had ideas of its own and it struck with a vengeance. I had not predicted that I would be so actively, violently ill every single day. For the first time in my life, there was something that dictated my day-to-day activities that I could not control. My style of learning had involved attending lectures, but this was abruptly halted as my morning sickness set in to stay. I was unable to keep my composure for extended periods of time, especially during three-hour-long gross anatomy dissections. There were days where I needed to stay home and take study break naps. Most days, I just wanted to function, which was difficult to accomplish. I tried to act as normal as possible because I didn't want any special treatment or to draw any special attention, even on days when I was miserable.

Thankfully, I wasn't always miserable. While there were plenty of doubts, there was even more joy. Seeing the ultrasounds, hearing the heart beat, learning that our baby was a girl, trying to decide on a name — all of these things were joyful, and I was grateful for something outside of school to help me feel like I wasn't completely consumed in my life as a medical student.

However, the problem with secrets is that eventually they reveal themselves. Concealing my pregnancy was no easy feat. One of our assignments for first year was an eight-hour shadowing shift in our university's emergency department, which was exceptionally busy that night. My assigned shift was during my period of extreme morning sickness, but there was no way to reschedule my shift without breaking my news to the administration. To keep my nausea at bay, I kept a large quantity of hard candies in my short white coat pocket. When there was a need for an x-ray, I quietly excused myself to a safe distance. The attending I was shadowing took notice, smiled at me, and returned to her work.

While my secret was safe that night, it was not to last. Not long thereafter, gross anatomy precipitated my decision to speak with my professors about my pregnancy. My stomach needed substance constantly, which meant I had to learn how much food to take with me to campus so I could be productive without too many breaks. I simply could not stay at my dissection table for long enough periods without having fresh air and a drink or a snack to settle my stomach, and I didn't want to be accused of trying to shirk my responsibilities at the dissection table. Over winter break, I was into the second trimester of my pregnancy, the nausea was slowly subsiding, and my husband and I had a clear ultrasound of a healthy baby. It was finally time to share our good news.

To my surprise, my classmates and my institution were wonderfully supportive over the course of my pregnancy. When it was no longer a secret from anyone, I quickly realized that all of my fears were unfounded. It was such a relief to no longer hide a major part of my life from those around me. Speaking to the administration also provided me with a long list of mentors in a variety of specialties who also started families while in school or early in their careers, which made me feel much less isolated in my experience. The most encouraging thing I gained from my mentors was hearing how their stories and experiences turned out, and that this was a much more common experience than I had anticipated.

While the nausea did finally subside, other things that I did not expect appeared. The small, day-to-day things that I could no longer do for myself started to feel like a betrayal. I could no longer bend over to tie my own shoes, so I bought slip-ons. My clothes were constantly getting tighter. Even reaching things on shelves became difficult, as my growing abdomen would get in the way. When the baby would kick during exams, my concentration would break and I would need a moment to refocus. When the long walk from the parking garage to campus became too much for me, I started taking the shuttle and had to factor in extra time to make the trip into campus.

Other things that I did not consider: timing. I had failed the one-hour GTT (glucose tolerance test) and then had to schedule a three-hour GTT to make sure I did not have gestational diabetes. Finding a convenient three-hour block of time to be absent from coursework and exams was tricky. These were all minor inconveniences but took some time to get used to as my new normal.

When thinking about starting a family during medical school, it can seem like an insurmountable task. There were many things that I wish I would have known and thought about before trying to start a family during my first year. Even though my pregnancy was much more difficult than I expected, the experience itself was not as horrible as it could have been. I attribute this to the support I received from my husband, family, classmates, and school administration — my self-consciousness was a burden that I placed upon myself that was unnecessary.

At the beginning, I was not sure that the outcome would be as happy as it has been; in hindsight, having a baby during medical school was not a bad idea at all.

Questions

1. How do you think pregnancy and parenthood affect medical training and vice versa?

2. How is parenthood different for males and females in medicine?

3. Do you think the way pregnancy and parenthood are treated in the medical community has an impact on retention of female physicians in the workforce?

4. At what point along the timeline of medical training is it optimal to start a family?

—Nikki Nametz Feinberg

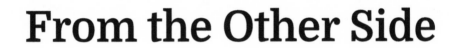

From the Other Side

For Pappou: A Reflection on Loss During the Clinical Years

April 8, 2013

Chris Meltsakos
New York Medical College
Class of 2014

IT WAS JUST A WEEK into our third-year rotations and my class was eagerly awaiting our Step 1 scores while adjusting to the beginnings of our clinical responsibilities. When the day came that our scores were to be released, I received a phone call from my aunt who told me that my Pappou (grandfather), who was in Greece on his yearly summer trip, had collapsed on his veranda and was en route to a local hospital. Immediately, hundreds of different diagnoses popped into my head as I worried about everything from his diabetes to the possibility of a stroke.

Later that evening, my aunt called back to update me about the situation. Physicians at the local hospital believed that my Pappou had a subarachnoid hemorrhage. But, because they didn't have a CT machine at the hospital, they were going to send him to another local hospital to confirm the diagnosis. In the meanwhile, my father and uncle were booking tickets to try to get to Greece as soon as possible.

I anxiously awaited another phone call and, around 8:30 p.m., my aunt called back. She informed me that they had rushed my Pappou to Thessaloniki, the nearest large city, because the smaller hospitals were not equipped to handle a subarachnoid bleed. She then broke the news to me that he had passed away shortly after his arrival. She told me that my uncle had received a phone call from the hospital while he and my father were sitting on the tarmac awaiting takeoff.

There was a long pause and I held back my tears. My Pappou and I were very close. This was a surreal and wrenching moment. As we both cried for a few minutes, I got off the phone to answer a call from my mother who had called to bear the same bad news. Even the second time around it did not seem real. I then took on the responsibility of calling my younger sister to let her know. It was a day that I'll never forget.

After experiencing alternating anger and sadness for about an hour, I quickly realized that this was just the beginning of what would be a long and difficult ordeal. I knew that it was going to be hard to get the body back to the United States, but that it would be even harder to afford the time off from my first clerkship to travel to Massachusetts to adequately mourn and be there with my family for the wake, the funeral and visitors.

I was correct in my thinking. It took us nearly 10 days to get my Pappou home, and I knew I couldn't feasibly take more than a day or two off from the clerkship, so we scheduled the wake for a Friday and the funeral the next day. Being the first-born grandchild and the closest to my grandparents, I wrote a eulogy in honor of my Pappou that I shared during the traditional Greek fish dinner that followed the funeral.

Although my story is not a story of patient interaction, or of an experience on the wards, this whole experience exemplifies the intricate connection between our work and our lives. Those of us in the health care profession have entered into a field that requires us to make many sacrifices, whether it be late nights, weekends or holidays. Experiencing the loss of my Pappou, while learning to balance this magnitude of work, was a difficult task. I was not able to spend as much time with my family as I would have liked during these difficult times, but the responsibility we take on as young physicians is extensive. We are required to make these sacrifices to help improve and save the lives of others.

I can certainly say that I've seen myself grow as an individual and as a young physician over these past few months. My time management, leadership skills and even interpersonal relationships have blossomed with each history and physical. I am no longer lost and uncomfortable in my short white coat. Rather, I am able work my way into any health care team in a "well-oiled" manner. My clinical experiences have shown me what it is to take care of another human being while remaining a devoted family member and good friend to others. I wanted to share this story as a story of loss in medicine because familial losses are just as trying as the losses we experience in the clinic and because our struggles in dealing with such matters overlap with our clinical duties.

The following is my eulogy to my Pappou. Although difficult to read again, I wanted to share it with the readers of *in-Training* in honor of the lessons he taught me and his undying pride and support of my medical career.

—

From July 23, 2012 — For Pappou

Before I share with all of you some of my thoughts, I'd like to share the words of a Ralph Waldo Emerson poem that I remembered reading in high school entitled "To laugh often and much."

To laugh often and much;
to win the respect of the intelligent people
and the affection of children;
to earn the appreciation of honest critics
and endure the betrayal of false friends;
to appreciate beauty;
to find the best in others;
to leave the world a bit better
whether by a healthy child,
a garden patch, or a redeemed social condition;
to know that one life has breathed easier because you lived here.
This is to have succeeded.

Why did I want to start with this poem? Well, written and spoken language remain inadequate to express the whirlpool of emotions that the human mind and soul may experience, but this poem at least serves as a starting point to discuss the magnitude of Pappou's contributions to our lives. From the time I was very little, Pappou had always shown me how to succeed. Whether it was putting a smile on my face while playing with my sister and I during childhood or, more recently, the way he would sit me down over lunch to talk with me about my goals in life and the "paths that lay before me," Pappou always wanted to instill within me the power to succeed.

Though his words, carefully chosen and perpetually succinct, offered great insight into his philosophies, it was Pappou's presence that seemed to have the most profound effect on me. Pappou was the kind of person you could quietly sit next to on a veranda for hours and not speak a word with, but remain in a state of mutual understanding and appreciation for the world and the details that surround us that words cannot capture. I can recall many of these moments over my lifetime, but the most powerful moments come from the summer of 2005 that I spent with Yia Yia and Pappou in Greece. I often think back to those moments spent sitting out on the balcony in the afternoon, either before or after some *mezedes*, just looking down at the garden below and the river just beyond. I remember simply taking in the details, sights, sounds and smells and appreciating the comforting presence of Pappou next to me, while simultaneously chuckling in my head at Yia Yia yelling at us to get into the shade. I am grateful for the evenings spent with Pappou sipping Greek coffee or frappe at the *"Pappoudes" Kaffenio* (grandfather's coffeehouse). Through his silent observation of the world around us during these moments, he taught me that we should not be alive, yet blind to the life we are living, but rather that we should celebrate life and appreciate the moments we can capture.

To me, this short time period marked the most personal growth that I've experienced in my life to this date. It was a period of time marking my growth from adolescence to young adulthood. I strengthened a relationship with my Yia Yia and Pappou that brought me closer to each of them than I could have possibly imagined. It was after this experience that I truly came to appreciate the etiology of the word "grandparents." Our forefathers were wise in their careful selection of language, because grandparents are nothing but a second set of parents. They are there to help love you, nurture you, and to assist you in your development to the best of their ability. It's unfortunate that, far too often in modern society, we forget this. Too many times we don't appreciate the depth of love, knowledge, and experience that our elders offer. I am so grateful for having realized this in my youth and for making the most of my relationships.

Pappou's careful observation of the world around him oftentimes went unnoticed. At Christmas or *Pasxa* (Easter), I would routinely glance over at Pappou, either sitting at the head of the table or by the *arni* (lamb), intently and proudly watching and listening. He would briefly offer his input in conversations and then return to that state of profound pride and observation. From the time I was about 14 years old, each year at Pasxa, it was almost an unsaid rule that I would help Pappou to cut the lamb and clean the *souvles* (kebab skewers) after. I loved these moments because, as we worked in unison, oftentimes after the others had brought the food inside, I was able to spend one on one time with Pappou, watching, learning, and listening in the same fashion he demonstrated by his careful enjoyment and observation of the world around him.

Pappou fostered and taught me much over the course of my life, and I'm so grateful for everything he has done for me. His passing marks one of the most difficult days of my life, because there was so much more that I was hoping to give back to him. I was looking forward to making him proud upon my medical school graduation, or sharing smiles with him on a wedding day, and even one day introducing a great-grandchild to him because I know these would be the most profound and valuable gifts I could offer for all of the knowledge, love, care and pride he'd shown to me throughout my life.

But we cannot dwell on what could be or on the plans we intended, for life is as much a mystery as death is. We must take solace in knowing that Pappou lived a long life full of love, care, pride, and happiness. I am forever grateful for making sure that I was never too "busy" for a phone call or lunch date. I am forever grateful for the kind of man I have become, in part due to the lessons of my Pappou.

Though Pappou may not be here with us in the physical realm, he is far from absent. He lives on in each and every one of us: in memory, in thought, in lessons and laughs. The greatest gift we can offer to Pappou is to celebrate his life and to try to embody his hard work, dedication, passion, love, kindness, and perpetual appreciation for the world around him each and everyday.

So as we weep and mourn the loss of a great man, I figured I'd part with a final quote by Washington Irving that is more than fitting at this point:

"There is sacredness in tears. They are not the mark of weakness, but of power. They speak more eloquently than ten thousand tongues. They are messengers of overwhelming grief … and unspeakable love."

Questions

1. Have you ever struggled to balance family responsibilities with medical school responsibilities? Were you able to balance the two? If so, what resources helped you achieve a balance? If not, why did you choose one over the other, and what barriers prevented you from achieving balance?

2. The author's inclusion of his grandfather's eulogy in this narrative not only honors the life of his grandfather, but also demonstrates how the author processed his grief — through writing. What strategies do you use for self-care in medical school?

3. The author's experience of loss gave him a stronger appreciation for the trials that patients and families in our care may be facing. How have your own personal struggles or challenges influenced your role as a medical student?

4. How would you aid a colleague who is going through a difficult time in his or her life?

5. The author describes his grandfather as an important source of support in his life. What people in your life are your supports? How do you or will you maintain those relationships during your time in medical school?

—Phyllis Ying

Medical Student as Patient

September 13, 2013

Lorenzo Sewanan
Yale School of Medicine
MSTP-3

S NOW AND FROST sculpted mazes in the streets; I struggled through the wind, fluid freezing in my joints, unpaved sidewalk sliding below my shoes. I was skating on a pond in Transylvania; the desolate snowscape wrapped around the hill crowned with the dark building, speckled but starkly rising. Maybe there were vampires in there, but my hands tingled with warmth as I opened the metal handles.

The guard glanced but said nothing. I felt immediately lost; words soliciting directions died in my throat. At one end of the vestibule, elevators chimed. A few seconds later, I followed a woman in blue scrubs and pink sneakers zigzagging through the third floor rooms. I did not get a chance to look at her, so I kept my eyes on the shoes; they directed me when she failed to do so vocally. Suddenly ceasing to move, she gestured strongly as she almost pushed me into a room. It was very much like the ones we used for practice, but this time, it would not be practice.

I sat on the padded table instead of the chair; it seemed more comfortable. I watched snow begin to fall, and my eyes started to wander. The ophthalmoscope seemed familiar in its steel and black plastic, but the size was larger than usual, and the metal more chrome than my faded secondhand instrument. In fact, everything in the office seemed used but spotless, even the hand sanitizer dispenser. I sat alone for a very long time.

She walked in then, bright-toothed smile topped by wide black glasses, stylish but professional. "Hi, Lorenzo. I'm Alice, and I'm your nurse practitioner today. What brings you in today? How are you feeling?"

I struggled to find the right words. "I am doing okay. I am..." She encouraged with a smile. Should I say I have trouble breathing, and I'm coughing, have pain when I breathe, and a sore throat? Or, should I say I think I have a lobar pneumonia of the right upper lobe, with common cold viral co-infection? "I'm having a hard time. I'm coughing and my throat hurts."

She said some irrelevant comforting words. She probably did not actually care; we are all taught to say these things to comfort the patient and make them more compliant. But, that in itself was warming; she was treating me like any other patient. Perhaps, she did not know?

Alice, the nurse practitioner, asked me to take off my shirt, and I did as she asked. Starting with my face, she palpated, searching for tenderness and lymph nodes, with fingers far more nimble and certain than mine ever were. From point to point, she listened to lungs, auscultating the L-shaped pattern on my back and my chest. "Your lungs are clear actually, so it's probably not anything serious like pneumonia."

I tried to look as if I'd never heard of pneumonia before. In fact, I started to think that she did not really know or if she knew, she did not show it.

"Pneumonia is an infection of the lungs, but you don't have that." She said it slowly and certainly, reassuring me of her ignorance.

"So what do you think it is?" I asked more loudly, wanting her attention instead of trying to avoid it.

"You most likely just have strep throat, which is an infection of the throat. It is easily treated. You don't have to worry. I'll just give you some antibiotics, and take a bit of your sputum to the lab. Here, take this and go spit in it at the sink."

I hawked up the deepest reserves of phlegm I could find, the thickest I could get, and I filled the little plastic sample vial up with green spit and handed it to her. It was her problem, not mine.

"Okay, just take this prescription and get these antibiotics. Take them three times a day, and I'll call you tomorrow with the results to let you know whether you should come in or not."

I shook her hand and left the room as quickly as possible after putting on my shirt. I'd never been happier to walk into a blizzard.

She had treated me like a normal person and not a medical student.

Questions

1. If you have been to the doctor while in medical school, was your experience different compared to before you were a medical student? Why do you think the experience was different?

2. How can being a patient make us better at being physicians? Has being a patient led to any changes in how, as a physician, you plan to treat patients?

3. "I'd never been happier to walk into a blizzard. She had treated me like a normal person, and not a medical student." What do you think the author means by this, and why do you think the author feels this way? Would you rather your health care provider know that you are a medical student? Why or why not?

—Vikas Bhatt

When a Patient's Disease Strikes a Chord

February 24, 2014

Anjani Amladi
The Commonwealth Medical College
Class of 2015

A FTER ARRIVING AT THE HOSPITAL, scrubbing in and warming up with a few anatomy questions with my attending, I was relaxed and ready to assist with the upcoming thyroidectomy. My patient, who will be referred to as "M," was a 17-year-old girl who presented to the office with dizziness. After an extensive workup it was discovered that her symptoms were due to thyroid dysfunction. The surgery was meant to be a straightforward case, but the next few hours were far from routine.

The first steps of the surgery went beautifully; however, while attempting to remove the first hemilobe of the thyroid, the surgeon saw something he did not quite expect. There was a growth that did not resemble normal tissue. The lobe was removed and sent to pathology STAT. The results: papillary thyroid carcinoma.

My knees buckled, my shoulders tensed and a surge of adrenaline ran through me. I was 24 years old when I was diagnosed with this very same disease.

The difficult part for me was the fact that prior to surgery M had no idea she had cancer. What made it even worse was the realization that when she woke up, someone was going to have to deliver the news.

Hours later when it came time to check on her I was scared. What happens if I get there and nobody told her? What happens if she does not want to see me? What happens if her parents are angry? All of these thoughts were circulating in my mind and I could not process them all at once.

When I finally got to her room, I was terrified but I knew seeing her was the right thing to do. I knocked on the door and was greeted by M and her mother. I introduced myself, asked how she was feeling and if there was anything she needed before I asked the looming question. "So, were you informed as to how your surgery went and the outcome?" She looked down, dropped her eyes and replied, "The surgery went fine, but they told me I have cancer."

I gently explained to her the reason it was so important for me to see her. I told her that two years ago, I too was diagnosed with the same kind of cancer she has. I told her that despite my diagnosis I am still successfully working toward my lifelong dream of becoming a physician, that I didn't lose any part of myself and that after surgery and radiation I am cancer free and am living a very healthy and happy life.

She looked up at me with tears in her eyes and said, "Thank you. The only other person in my family I know of who had cancer died almost immediately after being diagnosed. I don't know how this happened, or why. And I can't stop crying. Sometimes I'll be laughing, like when I talk to my sister and then I just cry for no reason at all." I told her she was entitled to feel however she wanted to about her diagnosis and explained that although sometimes bad things happen to good people, she would still be able to live the life she always dreamed of. After deciding she needed to get some rest, I promised to check on her in the morning, and said goodnight.

When I walked in the next day she was happy to see me and she looked much better than the night before. I sat down and talked to her for a while, gave her a hug, my contact information and wished her well. I was standing in front of the elevator on my way out and when the doors opened I saw M's mother. She immediately greeted me with a smile and a hug and told me that after my visit, she and her husband were so grateful and were filled with hope instead of fear. She said that M felt much better about her diagnosis, and that they will be forever grateful for what I had done. I told her I was so appreciative that my visits made a difference and said that I did what I thought was right and was glad it helped. She hugged me again and with tears in her eyes, said goodbye and proceeded to her daughter's room.

It took me several days to really absorb and reflect on the patient encounter I had and it helped me come to terms with my own illness experience. Getting to know M was a blessing because in my talks with her, I was able to provide reassurance, comfort and a shoulder to lean on from the unique perspective of being a survivor of the same illness. In a way, providing guidance and support to her was not only healing for her but also for me. My experience with her reminded me that the healing process does not end simply when interventions are completed. The doctor-patient relationship extends far beyond that.

The patient encounter is part of the healing process too and it's important to be reminded of that. Kind words, a caring demeanor and authentic acts are as much a part of the healing process as any physical intervention we could offer. This experience not only reaffirmed my reasons for wanting to become a doctor, but it also helped me add a silver lining to my very traumatic illness experience. This experience helped me become a better medical student, a better person and will no doubt help me become a better doctor. It is an experience I will remember and cherish always and am grateful to have been a part of it.

Questions

1. The author describes how her experience with a disease affected her feelings toward a patient with the same disease. Has this ever happened to you and, if so, how did it affect how you cared for the patient? If not, discuss a past life experience of your own that may affect your relationship with a future patient.

2. Is there a risk in self-disclosure to a patient? How might this affect the doctor-patient relationship? Could it have a positive effect or a negative effect, and why?

3. What are some of your own fears about your future medical career? How will you overcome the desire to run away and continue to do the "right thing"?

4. Sharing experiences with patients, as in this story, may allow us to connect with our patients in a way that few others can. Discuss any experiences you have had in the past with patients or people outside of medicine in which you were able to connect through shared experiences. Why is it that shared experiences bring people into special relationships?

5. The author describes how this encounter with her patient allowed her to revisit her past experience with thyroid cancer and "come to terms" with it. As physicians and health care providers, we are in a special position to impact the lives of our patients, but it is also true that they may profoundly impact our own lives. Discuss.

—Chris Deans

Parenthesis
March 28, 2014

Amanda Rutishauser
Michigan State University College of Human Medicine
Class of 2016

It was a Thursday in November,
a day that felt like neither Thursday nor November
a few weeks after my diagnosis
that hadn't seemed quite right, either,
and here it was, on the page:
the perfect trap, the perfect analogy.

The patient (My Name

No closing parenthesis.

Now perhaps you're one of those people
who thinks that a missing closing parenthesis is just another typo,
like a comma too few or too many.
Perhaps you've yet to realize that the greatest danger
facing any reader is an open parenthesis with no end.

My medical record. My diagnosis. My trap.
For the rest of my life, it seemed, I would be tucked under the arm
of that parenthesis, the two of us, me a forever aside, a soliloquy,
nevermore myself.

I crossed the street from the hospital to the parking garage.
It was rush hour traffic and a white van scraped by me
like a leaf over a frozen pond.
I barely felt it, safe as I was behind my parenthesis,
like a cold, glass lens
that protected and magnified me
not into something greater but made me larger
with no more density — only diluted.

The patient, my name, the great divide.
I felt like a goldfish in its bowl,
an expansive bowl like an ocean
yet swim to the very edge and there's nothing
but that smooth curve of glass — (
the world goes on outside yet here I am
all to myself in my aquarium,
my world and the world I see
forever separate.

Diagnosis or open parenthesis: which the greater evil?
Both had upon me the same effect and yet it was easier
to understand myself in terms of the parenthesis —
a parenthetical infinity that I had entered —
than to believe there was no barrier but that inside me.
My heart, my ovaries, my liver, my lungs,
each once cupped in () now just (

))

Questions

This poem was written by the author assuming the point of view of a patient
she had cared for. What are the benefits of stepping into someone else's
shoes in this way? What are the dangers?

—Aleena Paul

Patient Autonomy: A Medical Student's Experience as a Patient

July 1, 2014

Crystal Romero
George Washington University School of Medicine
Class of 2018

*M*S. ROMERO IS AN *otherwise healthy medical student who was transferred to the MICU with acute liver failure; isoniazid toxicity. Crystal had a positive PPD screening, negative chest x-ray and started therapy for potential LTBI. After seven weeks the patient felt fatigued, anorexic, jaundiced, RUQ abdominal pain, and was found to have elevated LFT's & INR. She was originally admitted to INOVA for observation, but was transferred to Medstar Georgetown University Hospital MICU and worked up for a possible liver transplant.*

My medical adventure was one of triumphs and failures on behalf of the medical profession. I would like to introduce three points I learned from this experience as both a patient and as a medical student. One of my first words of advice is: don't assume that a patient doesn't fit the criteria for a medical condition purely because you "think" it is unlikely. Four weeks into treatment I sought medical care for abdominal pain and was sent away without blood work, even when I questioned if I was having a reaction to the isoniazid. Two weeks later my symptoms intensified and had been turned away again. A few days passed after that, I sought medical care from the ER and was sent home twice; my INR was not assessed. The ER doctor even had the gall to quiz me on Prometheus, a tale of a man whose liver is eaten by a crow, and dismissed my pain because, as I should have learned, the liver regenerates.

Then the battle truly began. Two days after my ER visit I was in the ICU preparing my family and myself for many possibilities, including liver transplant and possible death. Although it had already been several days since I had stopped the medication on my own, my LFT's and INR were trending upwards. If it had not been for the GI doctor I had never met, I would not be alive today. Only knowing me by looking at lab data and trends that signified that I was in liver failure, he called my personal cell and admitted me to the hospital.

Second, every patient is a person first and foremost. Every physician is also a person; humanity is an inherent trait. Throughout this battle I've had medical personnel trivialize my fight for life by treating and speaking to me with utter disrespect. However, I am the only one who must live with the long-term physical ramifications health-wise. At one point, the physician responsible for the neglect accused me of being an excessive drinker to cover up her errors; however, this empty accusation was proven unfounded.

On the other hand, I have also seen the beauty of medicine. Nurse Ashley, one of the nurses in charge of bathing me, was quintessential to the restoration of my faith in humanity, as well as medicine. Although I lay infirm and ready to die, she spoke to me while looking in my eyes as she bathed me and allowed me to wipe the most intimate areas of my body in an attempt to maintain my dignity. She chatted with me about sports I played, shows I watched and my passions — the things that made me human. In another instance, I was taken by surprise when one of the residents came to visit me on his day off, held my hand, and spoke to me about his own medical adventure. The compassion and respect that I felt from some medical professionals reminded me of the innate humanness we possess as both patients and as physicians.

Third, never assume that the patient is at fault for his or her pain and never treat him or her like it is. Some of the stigma associated with liver disease haunted me as the follow-up's piled and the number of specialists added up. One nurse commented during a follow-up visit while performing blood draw, "You have really been enjoying life." She had already formulated an opinion that I was a drug addict or alcoholic, never stopping to think that maybe this was not my own doing. On the other hand, my team of doctors in charge of my recovery lifted my spirits when they praised me for having been as good to my body as I had before, during and after this debacle. In fact, they reminded me that had I participated in any of these pastimes I would have likely passed away.

Physicians practice in the hope of doing less harm than good. When medical practice becomes automatic and sterile, the profession needs an overhaul. It's unfortunate that a few negligent physicians are representative of medicine as a whole to the public because as the patient, it leaves a bitter taste in my mouth. However, as a future physician, it empowers me to trust myself and to never have blind faith in the constantly evolving field of medicine. For the physicians responsible for the medical neglect in my case, medicine had become rote — hence the shortcuts in my level of care. The physicians initially in charge of my care failed me when they put me on a medication known to cause liver failure and never checked my liver function, even when I presented with classical symptoms. They failed to follow the Hippocratic Oath to do no harm.

Alternatively, I've witnessed a sense of camaraderie, compassion and affection from physicians and nurses I would never have known otherwise, that have helped keep me from deterring from my chosen career path. Nurse Jan was both stern and compassionate with my mother when she lost her composure at the first sight of her eldest child hooked to several machines with IVs running in every direction. She looked at my mother and said, "You have to be strong." At the end of the day, I have no ill-will against the "profession of medicine" and I look forward to being a great physician.

Questions

1. What do you think makes doctors forget that their patients are people?

2. The author states that when medical practice becomes "automatic and sterile," it is time for the profession of medicine to change. Have you witnessed a situation in which medical practice was automatic or sterile? How do you think the profession of medicine can change that type of medical practice?

3. How would you have responded to the nurse who assumed that the author had abused drugs and alcohol? Would you have set her straight or remained silent?

4. Discuss the doctors and nurses who had a positive impact on the author and her family. Was it only their actions that had an impact, or their words, too? Do you need both?

5. Describe a situation where you were the patient and you felt mistreated, or you witnessed a patient being mistreated. What happened? How can you prevent yourself from treating a patient this way?

—Melanie Watt

Treating the Disease and Treating the Illness

October 1, 2014

Steven Lange
Albany Medical College
Class of 2017

STANDING AT THE FOOT of her hospital bed, it was clear to me — as it was to the attending physician — that my grandmother was suffering from a disease: an obvious structural disorder identified by scientific medicine as negatively impacting her health. *Hilar mass, cavitation, hypercalcemia. Keratin pearls, intercellular bridges. Hemoptysis, dyspnea, edema.*

It was also apparent to this eight year-old, however, that she was burdened by an *illness*, or an impaired sense of well-being. *She was bedridden, depressed, solemn. She lost her beautiful hair, her clear voice, her levity.* The disease existed regardless of her knowing, but her illness thrived in her conscience.

My grandmother's lung cancer was being treated by the best physicians trained by the nation's top institutions and armed with modern technology. Her illness, that set of subjective experiences and feelings which helped her cope with cancer, relied not on this specific expertise, but on a compassion which came from an understanding of her private hardship.

I waited there in naïve wonder, pondering loaded questions. Why did my grandmother suffer? What did it mean to be a patient? What could be done to support her, physically and emotionally?

When we think about disease, we often rely on definitions rooted in physiology. This classification is pragmatic and beneficial, allowing physicians to perform their work with attention to biological schema. On a greater scale, however, disease encompasses the entirety of the individual by framing identity and altering perception. Disease is as much cultural as it is chemical, and as historical as it is personal. The Oxford English Dictionary describes disease primarily as "discomfort, inconvenience." First recorded in the early 14th century, a hiatus in human history between the Middle Ages and the Renaissance, ravished by the Little Ice Age and the Black Plague, the word "disease" came to be a signpost for general conflict between person and nature. Disease soon acquired the essence of sickness in the latter half of the century, and was understood to be *disorder*: a distasteful bodily feeling that was symptomatologically manifest. Though "disease" expanded its definition with time, acquiring more modern dressings adorned by Enlightenment-era natural science, it continued to retain the foundational sense we might now name "unease." Disease represents the abnormal conditions and adverse events which change its victim's habitus, and is used by today's physicians as an objective diagnostic term.

The central idea of illness is, however, an ancient concept that invokes religious and moral themes. One of the earliest mysteries which humankind sought to explain, illness — innately malevolent, morally wrong and unpleasantly uncertain — entered our collective consciousness epochs before scientific medicine, whose influence nonetheless will likely supersede that of its predecessors. The earliest ideas of medicine and health were intimately tied with religion, as still persists today despite growing scientific knowledge. Early Chinese medicine and that of the Old Testament shared a supernatural belief about illness, which was explained by a fate controlled by external forces, players or spirits. A body of Sanskrit literature, the Veda, contains prayers of health to the gods who were believed to have healing powers over evil entities that disrupted three bodily "humors," comparable to Hippocrates' estimation of four humors: black bile, yellow bile, blood and phlegm.

The development of scientific thinking in Greece, however, competed with the prevalence of mythological belief. Many non-Western theories of illness also grew under the guise of predominating beliefs and often melded with them, often influencing human behavior by shaping the idea of (and creating meaning for) an unknown disease.[1] The changing landscape of disease evolved concurrently with advances in human thinking, though misrepresentation and misinterpretation were omnipresent. Our basic responses to the nature of disease and the meaning of nature compelled our ancestors to devise both reasonable and unreasonable explanations to corporeal phenomena. Still today, we use metaphor as a device for understanding disease and illness. Our perceptions of both disease and illness allow us to identify, treat and think about them.

A skim through "Harrison's Principles of Internal Medicine" or the latest edition of the DSM gives a clear idea of disease as diverse, multiplicitous and informed by numerous fields. Disease is diagnosed and treated in a variety of manners, and differs from person to person. Though a disease can be universally accepted to follow a particular pattern, its specific course through an individual at any point in time is likely to take on a character of its own: a biological and psychological effect/affect which unifies the patient/subject and the disease/object. Illness is dynamic, following both top-down and bottom-up designs; it can define a person directly as well as be recast or redefined by one's emotion, perception and worldview. Basic beliefs about disease and one's relation to it constructs illness as a theme in an individual's life.

Illness can be thought of as a metaphor, which analogizes or associates a subject and an unrelated object. Illness refers to an abnormality that the subject may not identify as part of oneself; many who consider themselves diseased or ill feel that they contain a foreign pathogen or harbor a "foreignness," something exterior or unfamiliar which does not effectively characterize one's sense of self. Because we may see disease as "not us" or "other," we can ascribe it its own being. Illness largely relies on stigmata and vernacular, and is molded by the conceptions and expectations of both society and the individual. The way in which we speak about illness, as a whole and as parts, and the metaphysical contours we create for it give it simultaneous color and uncertainty. It becomes an emblematic homunculus, containing all the ideas — true and false, scientific and religious, causative and caused — that render its caricature. While disease may depend on signs and symptoms, illnesses rely on mood and metaphor for communication, as many ideas are wont to do.

Disease and illness are often used interchangeably, and though they are descriptively different they are embedded in a common dialogue. Illness compels the patient to seek medical attention, but the disease is what prompts treatment. The emergent qualities which culminate in an illness do not always reflect the internal disease; what exists in the eyes, ears and hands of an astute physician is not always what is felt or experienced by the patient. Disease provides the raw materials with which illnesses are sculpted. Disease, however, has benefitted from modern advancements in medicine while illness has retained the characteristics which have conceptualized human suffering for years. Thus, though we can more accurately identify and treat diseases that our fathers and grandfathers could not, in many cases we pictorialize and react to them in traditional, conditioned ways.

The physician is rightly trained to regard infirmity as a physical transgressor whose actions must be controlled. From the physician's point of view, disease is a tangible task. To the patient, the disease is a pressing problem. To the physician, the illness is sometimes a hindrance to diagnosis and treatment while to the patient it is a characteristic burden that can be duly informative. To the patient, the illness may be more real than the disease, for though the disease governs physiology the illness directs the patient's psychosocial behavior. The physician, however, understands that the underlying issue must be assessed before any improvement can be considered. Even so, an open-minded approach to both disease and illness is warranted. Because they are not mutually exclusive, disease and illness can be simultaneously addressed in the management of a patient. The disease may be detectable only by the physician, while the illness is reportable by the patient. The attitudes of the physician and patient should be made compatible in order to effect an optimal approach to medical care. The distinction between *being* and *feeling* sick, and an attention to what causes *death* versus *suffering*, can reconcile the oft confused relationship between disease and illness.

Illness has historically been seen as an expression of character: something intimately tied to a person's being and representative of their thoughts, actions and beliefs. It has long been felt as a way for the body to describe itself: how the disease in question is construed in the totality of the person. Explaining illness solely in terms of disease is a reductionist constraint which neglects the complexity and threatens the quality of human life. Sometimes, a patient may have an asymptomatic disease, in which a disease is present without producing illness. Likewise, there are many patients who experience particular symptoms which are unable to be explained by disease. Two individuals with the same disease may also report different illnesses, a result perhaps justified by minor differences in physiology, cultural variables and "extremes of stoicism [which] often contribute tragically to delay and noncompliance."[2] Nonetheless, is it in the best interest of the physician and the patient to communicate these ramifications of sickness.

My grandmother needed the qualification of her illness as something particular to her: something which struck the entirety of her being, affected the whole of her person, a cause of suffering that influenced her quality of life. It is dissatisfying to be labeled with a disease, and difficult to adjust to the changes it brings. It is difficult to anticipate with full guarantee the presentation of a disease in a person. Both the well-controlled and poorly managed disease requires the care and attention that extends beyond the blood smear or CT, for there are aspects of sickness that are not concretely detectable or officially testable. Oftentimes, it is the illness which a patient wishes the physician to fix and which becomes the culprit of their disenchantment.

In that hospital room, I did my best to console the illness whose disease was being diligently managed by physicians, nurses and technicians. I did my best to remind my grandmother that she was a strong woman, and not a numbered carcinoma.

Questions

1. Think about a time when you cared for someone who had both a disease and illness. Did you note the distinctions discussed by the author?

2. What are some other terms and phrases we use in medicine that are a product of history?

—Aleena Paul

Broken

November 24, 2014

Jennifer Tsai
Warren Alpert Medical School of Brown University
Class of 2018

STRAIGHT ARMS. Lock elbows. Depress three to five centimeters down into the chest. Stay perpendicular to sternum. Keep rhythm. Do not relent.

"If you don't break ribs, you're not doing it right," my classmate jokes. He must know — he is one of three experienced paramedics in the classroom.

He has seen this all before.

"There is a high risk, during cardiopulmonary resuscitation, that the ribs will be broken." Our training pamphlet makes it clear. It is common clinical collateral — an expected expense.

A necessary evil.

There is a green, gated door in Kaohsiung, Taiwan that I have passed through since before I could walk. It is two blocks away from a small, dusty tributary overhung with bright red lanterns at all times of the year and three blocks away from a rather spontaneous-looking temple interweaved with elaborate dragons wrapped in golden scales. If you walk two blocks forward, three blocks left, take a right, and then a left, you will come upon a bustling market with some of the best street food you'll ever taste. It will be served from pots that are of questionable hygienic standards, slopped into old cracked bowls by ungloved hands, scooped with flimsy pink plastic spoons, and despite the cacophony of clucking chickens and aggressive bargaining, you will revel in every bite.

I do not know the names of these streets, or what to call the market, or who to pray to in the temple. I could not tell a traveler how to get there. I only know their locations in relation to the green door, in relation to the place where my father's family has lived and loved for decades. It is where we gather around a bowl of fat, seeded grapes, fresh *longyan*, slices of vibrant starfruit, and creamy wedges of guava. This green door has watched my father come home from elementary school, watched me return from America, watched my cousin as she left to be married. It has watched our family grow larger.

And now it has seen my family grow smaller.

Two days ago, my grandfather was found slumped outside the green door without a pulse. Two blocks from the weaving red lanterns, three blocks from the golden dragons, six blocks from the busy stalls with flimsy pink plastic spoons.

I imagine that the green door watched as the paramedics broke three of my grandfather's ribs in their attempt to save him.

A necessary evil.

Straight arms. Lock elbows. Depress three to five centimeters down into the chest. Stay perpendicular to sternum. Keep rhythm. Do not relent.

They tell the class that in our attempts of CPR, it is likely that ribs will snap beneath our one-and-two-and-three-and rhythm. That while we hum "Staying Alive" to keep the beat of our compressions, we will oftentimes splinter the safeguards of the heart. We may not even realize what we have done. We will be spurred on by our adrenaline, by our inexperience, by our overzealous fervor to save a life. They tell us with a chuckle. They tell us like it is a rite of passage.

We listen in class as if our professors will tell us how to solve the mysteries of medicine. We study our books as if they will give us the answers to health and healing. We apply ourselves as if memorizing these facts will teach us how to be good doctors.

"If you don't break ribs, you're not doing it right."

My grandfather, at 89 years old, cannot take the pain of his bruised, cracked, and broken ribs. He promptly signs a DNR — Do Not Resuscitate. It is now unlawful for the doctors to try and save him if his heart stops again.

He does not imagine that opening his eyes one more time is worth waking up to more of this pain.

The doctors cannot fix what they have broken.

As I sit here, surrounded by lecture notes and anatomy atlases, flashcards and color-coordinated study guides, my parents are flying home to Taiwan. My father will enter that green door, but his father will not ever again. This is another loved one that I will not be able to say goodbye to because I cannot afford to leave school. This is the second grandfather that will pass while I am sitting at my desk miles and miles away.

"There is a high risk, during cardiopulmonary resuscitation, that the ribs will be broken."

It is unnerving to watch a creature crawl out of the pages of a book.

The last time I saw my grandfather, he was leaning on his cane, ushering me into a taxi. I can see the green door behind him.

He told me to study hard in medical school.

Questions

1. Whether it is the chemist's drug, the surgeon's knife, or the hands of the one resuscitating, how do we reconcile doing harm to our patients in order to do good?

2. In your pursuit of a medical career, what have you had to sacrifice? Family? Time? Love? Have you mourned these? Should you mourn?

3. In the midst of the sacrifice that is medical training, it is easy to forget all those who have inspired you along the way. Who in your life has pushed you, challenged you and supported you? In what way do you believe you can honor them most?

—Eric Donahue

Systemic Afflictions

A Night at the Homeless Shelter

December 21, 2012

Jimmy Tam Huy Pham
Arizona College of Osteopathic Medicine
Class of 2015

TONIGHT IS NOT ANY DIFFERENT. A list of twenty-five patients to be seen. A standing room full of eager volunteer medical students — who just can't wait to do some doctoring — and a lone attending physician, a family physician who probably enjoys seeing the medical students acting important, walking around with their shiny stethoscopes around their necks, more than anything else.

On second thought, maybe the doctor is here every week because he wants to get away from his mundane morning office routine of patient check-ups. Whatever the reason is, he has been here for as long as I can remember, when I started volunteering at this shelter two years ago.

The brief instruction was announced. It's the usual: focused exams, presentation to the attending, well-thought assessments, and reasonable treatment plans. I was handed the first chart: "Here is your first patient. Go to work!"

"A white female in her fifties presented with..." *Heck, please skip the formalities! She is here because of pain!* They are all here because of pain! Pain in the knee joint. Pain in the lower back. Pain in the head, too. The kind that no medicine can cure.

"A white male presented with shotgun wound..." Yes, the one that he could die from — if that little copper thing changed direction just a few centimeters inward.

"A middle-aged Hispanic male complains of excruciating pain in the lumbar region of T3 through T6..." *Of course it is excruciating pain.* They never come in until the pain has worsened.

"A young white female presented with multiple complaints: nodule on tongue, pain in right knee, constant nasal discharge ... but chief complaint was an ingrown toenail..." *An ingrown toenail?* Yes, just an ingrown toenail!

Every day, they walk all morning and sleep all night. That's all these patients can do, anyways, besides working at menial jobs from week to week. They always seem to be in a hurry. *Where can you go? You are here for the night. You are here for treatment. Let me find out what is wrong with you.* They all seem to have a lot to tell. If you ask the right question and if you let them talk, they will tell you many things, everything.

Did I mention that the white female in her fifties has Crouzon syndrome? Yes, she had over twelve cranial surgeries and several more on her legs. She has three children: two boys who also have Crouzon and a daughter whose whereabouts she no longer knows. She has been bound to a wheelchair for years and weighs only eighty pounds.

And the white male with the shotgun wound. Well, he was agitated, shaken, angry, fidgeting, and asked me if he "could have done anything differently."

"What do you mean differently?"

"I could have known and fought back, couldn't I?"

"Let me look at your wound and see if I can do anything for you."

I did not answer his question. It could not be answered. There was no way it could be answered.

"Your wound is superficial."

My best diagnosis.

"What does that mean? Will it get infected? Will I die?"

"It's benign ... I mean, it looks real good. It will heal soon. Don't touch it with dirty hands, okay?"

Final assessment: debridement of pus, antibiotics, and stay away from dangerous neighborhoods!

The Hispanic man had a home and a good job. He was a truck driver. One day, he got beaten up really bad. Got hurt really bad in the shoulder and lower back. Could not work anymore. Now homeless. Been homeless for seven years — from Michigan, to California, now Arizona.

The young white female is a teenager. She no longer can stay in foster homes. She turned eighteen three weeks ago. The system says, "you are an adult now, go somewhere." So she goes here, the homeless shelter. Still a senior in high school. Not sexually active. *Differential of STD for that nodule in her mouth is out of the window!* No parents. Don't know who they are. Supposed to have some relatives somewhere but never spoke with them. Treated her for pain and educated on ingrown toenail. Then sent out on her way. Just like her foster parents did.

Tonight was just another night, not any different — for them.

For me, it is always different.

They told me their stories of resiliency and life. They lend me their body and sickness. They taught me the humanity of medicine.

Questions

1. How does the setting where health care is dispensed affect the patient-physician relationship?

2. Reflect on the social determinants of health that play a role in the stories of each of the patients described in this piece. How much impact did the author have on these patients' health?

3. Is it ethical that medical students are in essence the "primary care providers" for these patients?

4. Reflect on changes that have occurred in health care policy in recent years. Has enough progress been made to provide care for underserved populations?

—Aleena Paul

A Wait for the Bus:
A Solution for Wandering in Dementia

March 13, 2014

Katie Taylor
Icahn School of Medicine at Mount Sinai
Class of 2016

I'M SITTING IN A CLASS on dementia. The doctor is lecturing about the condition's prevalence, prognosis, neuropathology, diagnostic criteria, risk factors, deterministic genes and pharmacologic treatment. On a slide entitled "Non-pharmacologic Management," the doctor tells us that dementia often leads to wandering. Half of those who wander and are not found in 24 hours are found dead. To try to prevent patients from wandering far, some assisted living centers have installed fake bus stops. When their urge to roam strikes, they will end up on a fake bus bench, next to a fake bus sign on the retirement home lawn — a twisted "Waiting for Godot." We in the audience let out a collective slough of *whats?* and *reallies?* We cannot believe such a peculiar solution has been tried and proven.

After class, I look up the history of these phantom bus stops. The first was installed on the front courtyard of the Benrath Senior Center in Dusseldorf, Germany. The mean age of patients at the Benrath Senior Center is 84. Many have dementia. The house staff catches most of the patients en route to their wandering locales, but, before the implementation of the fake bus stop, if the travelers were determined and could not be convinced to stay, the center's only options were to lock them in their rooms or sedate them. Further, a few seniors had made it onto city buses. For example, in a fervent search for her long-dead mother, one patient had even made it back to her childhood home, only to find other people living in it.

We had learned in a previous lecture that short-term memory is the frailest of all memory types. The cerebral infiltrates of dementia dine first on the recent past, working backwards in time, leaving the younger self for last. After recent history has been consumed by memory loss, our brains choose to believe we have the homes, jobs and to-do lists from decades prior. Patients become stricken with an ostensible realization of who they are, and where they need to be, only to be confused when nurses stop them in the halls, and shake their heads no.

When escapees could not be found on the grounds, the center had to call the police. Phone calls with panicked family and manhunts ensued. Looking for a solution, the center began brainstorming, and eventually consulted a local care association, which suggested the fake bus stop. In a leap of faith in the unusual, the center persuaded the local transit authority to install an exact copy of a Dusseldorf city bus stop outside the center's front door, complete with the city's green and yellow bus stop sign, posted times, and a bench matching all the others in town. So convincing was the imitation that neighbors of the center started waiting at it for buses to arrive, until knowing nurses explained the get-up and shooed them away. The center staff waited to see if a patient would be so convinced.

A few days went by until a woman from the center insisted on seeing her young children. She was frantic and agitated and could not be convinced Benrath was her home and her children were grown. A nurse led her to the bus stop, and they sat down.

They listened to the birds, and felt the afternoon sun. They watched cars go by. Soon, the resident's panic receded. She forgot why she was there in the first place. The nurse invited her inside for coffee and the two walked back to the center. To forget you are in the present leads you to the past; to forget the past, leads you back to the present. In a double negative of amnesia, forgetfulness is the cure for forgetfulness.

Is it unkind to offer a partial omission of the truth — that no bus picks up at this stop? Do we owe the patients a dose of the hard facts? Or is it crueler to inflict a reality onto a patient that has a limited to no capacity to understand it? After reading how patients interact with the fake bus stop, the premise no longer felt Kafkaesque or deceitful to me — which it had felt somewhat when I first learned about it in class. Instead, the bus stop seems more like a welcoming twilight, where distinct realities can calmly and quietly ebb and flow. In the safe, liminal zone of the bus stop bench, patients can be any age and exist in any present, without staff forcing truth or medicine onto and into them. The director of the center says you cannot argue with these patients because they cannot rationally be convinced. "You have to deal with them in the reality in which they live," he says.

The Benrath bus stop is used every few days, now, either by those residents who get away without anyone noticing at first, or by those that have been led there, like the bench's first patient, to wait until the patient's urge to leave goes missing itself. The director says that the bus stop has changed how the staff approaches all residents — the staff has become more amenable to their patients' insistence, and consequently more readily make allowances for a patient's perceived reality. For example, prior to the stop, a retired baker kept waking and wandering at his old baking start-time. The staff would find him night after night in the kitchen at 2 a.m., frustrated nothing was set up for the day's bake, and each night, the staff would corral him back to his room. However, since the bus stop has been installed, the staff has decided to let him make a go of it, and now the patient is allowed to bake each morning.

The Benrath bus stop was so successful in managing patients with dementia that soon other senior centers in the city installed their own faux stops, and the idea spread across Germany, and soon, across Europe.

We learned in an earlier lecture on neurology that Alzheimer's is the leading cause of dementia, and that there are few medical interventions available to treat dementia. Unfortunately, scientists are not sure what causes Alzheimer's — they are just as confused as the patients are as to what is happening inside their brains. In fact, one cannot definitively diagnose Alzheimer's until the brain has been dissected. There is no cure. The disease causes continuous, progressive, irreversible cerebral damage until you die, which is on average five to 10 years after the diagnosis. Alzheimer's drugs help, but only somewhat. Doctors can mitigate the effects of dementia with donepezil or memantine, we learned in our pharmacology class, but they cannot prevent the disease's crippling progression. Once off the drugs, patients perform just as poorly on memory tests as those who had never taken Alzheimer's drugs at all.

Working with a problematic disease, an unknown etiology and medications that can mask the neural deterioration but cannot stop it, this thinking-out-of-the-box senior center designed a space — a treatment, really — that allowed their patients to explore their panic and pain, and let go of false realities. In all of its unlikeliness, their solution is stunning in its tragic-comedy, simplicity and genius. It does not fight the aging brain, but allows for it to *be*. It is non-invasive. There are no side effects, unless you count decreased mental anguish. It can be individualized. It is cost-effective. Lastly, it is practical and kind, all of which making the fake stop completely unlike most treatments for intractable diseases I have learned about in medical school so far.

Before moving on to the next slide, the lecturer mentioned that researchers think the wandering could also be a search for meaning. That is, not only are patients with dementia searching for their past, but they are trying to find a purpose they know has been lost, along with the health of their hippocampi and medial temporal lobes. What a testament to the aging human brain, that despite atrophy and invading debris, there perhaps remains a deep, underlying resolve to search for something more. I would like to believe that this hypothesis is true. In that way, I think octogenarians and scientists are cut from similar cloth — from confusion and non-understanding, springs a search for consequence.

Questions

1. Do you agree with the author's conclusions about the "fake bus stop"? Do you believe such interventions are worth the investment of resources?

2. Have you come across any other unconventional ideas and/or solutions to various medical problems? What are the challenges involved in implementing such ideas?

3. The last paragraph discusses wandering in dementia, and how it may be "a search for meaning." Do you agree, and why or why not?

4. Do you know anyone with Alzheimer's disease? If so, do you imagine that the "fake bus stop" may be helpful to that individual?

—Diane Brackett

How Health Care Policy Shapes Health Care Practice

June 24, 2014

Manasa Mouli
Tufts University School of Medicine
Class of 2015

THE PATIENT IS A 45-year-old man. When I enter the room with the resident, he is sitting on the edge of the exam table, wearing a poorly-constructed hospital gown. When I introduce myself, he struggles to keep on the paper garment while extending his hand towards mine. He is a pleasant man, overall, except for a lot of physical discomfort evident in his facial expressions.

The resident asks the patient about his symptoms. She asks whether the medication is working for him. Whether he has experienced aches. Whether he can walk, go to work. Whether the skin and joints of his arms, legs, trunk, face, palms, soles are healthy. The list goes on and on.

He tells us that, due to severe joint pain, he has not been able to drive much or work. He has stopped seeing his friends recently. His mood is low. He struggles to function in his normal routine, while experiencing constant pain. It is especially bad when he has flare-ups of his disease.

This patient has severe psoriasis. He also has depression, a commonly undiagnosed co-morbidity associated with this devastating autoimmune disease. He has had his disease since his early 20s. His initial presentation to the dermatology clinic marked the beginning of a battle involving his disease, his caregivers and his insurance company.

His doctor has recommended several topical steroids, which failed. She then switched him to phototherapy, which also failed. Currently he has been using methotrexate, and it is failing as well. The interesting point in this case is that the doctor knew the patient would fail methotrexate. The patient knew this too. She prescribed it because the insurance policy would not cover any other treatments until methotrexate had failed.

Later, she and I discussed this case. A great number of patients with moderate to severe plaque psoriasis, who have had their disease for many years without adequate response to other therapies, have been shown to significantly improve in response to ustekinumab, a biologic therapy. Biologic targeted therapy has shown greater efficacy than systemic and phototherapy in some patients. In this case, the doctor knew that based on this patient's presentation, history and symptoms, he would respond best to ustekinumab. She also knew that she could not prescribe it until the insurance company had been satisfied by trials of other treatments. It is a waste of time and resources, but unfortunately the protocol needs to be followed. When a doctor feels tied to the regulations of a third party, and the patient is bound to non-ideal treatment options, the health care system loses too. It is a waste of additional appointment slots, lab tests and administrative billing services.

And perhaps, we are providing substandard care. Our system is failing this patient. Policies are dictating the way doctors practice medicine and the choices patients are allowed to make.

I worked in the United Kingdom in an NHS-based system for a period of time. The combination of the National Health Service and the United Kingdom's welfare system means that the laws governing medical practice are very different there.

We had a patient who presented to the outpatient psychiatry unit, which specialized in eating disorders. She was a 23-year-old female (initially presenting at age 13) with a history of depression, sexual abuse, anorexia nervosa and numerous medical complications stemming from her psychiatric illness. Her other medical problems included osteoporosis, urinary incontinence, amenorrhea, liver failure and kidney failure.

Anorexia nervosa is a complicated disease to tackle, and this patient had been supported by social services since age 12. Her disease prevented her from being able to study, work or have a normal routine. After six years of ongoing therapy and numerous hospitalizations, she finally reached a stage where we could say that she was in "recovery." Although one can never fully recover from an eating disorder, it is possible to keep the disease under control and restore patients to normal function.

She started to take part-time classes several months before I met her. She had been steadily improving, with occasional lapses in her condition. For several months, the team of psychiatrists and nurses had been encouraging her to consider finding a part-time job. For some reason, each time this suggestion was seriously pursued, the patient became resistant to treatment and suffered from sudden binging and purging episodes.

One day I was chatting with her in the patient lounge. She seemed hesitant to accept praise and encouragement regarding the "normal" part of her life (her routine of class work), and when probed further about what triggered her binging habit, she became silent. I was about to leave the room when she blurted out the question pressing on her mind the most:

"Will I lose my disability benefits if I get a job? Suppose I really start to get better — does that mean I won't get that help that I need?"

I was stumped. On the one hand, it makes sense that if she were to reach the stage where her disease was under control and she was fully functional, she would no longer need to be on disability. On the other hand, who decides that point of recovery? The governing regulations have a cutoff point, where if a patient begins to recover, there is the strong possibility that she would immediately lose her benefits. However, without that extra support, there is a strong possibility that she will quickly relapse, especially under such severe financial constraints.

I spoke to more experienced staff members about this, and they expressed their disappointment at the system's failure to address this issue. By keeping patients financially constrained and incentivizing them to remain "unwell" (by the definition outlined in the regulation), again, it is the system that loses as a whole. Health care workers invest more time and money into care of patients who may be better managed in other ways. Patients start to lose their will to recover, something which is crucial in all medical care, but especially so in psychiatric illnesses.

These stories raise concerns about how much choice knowledge-empowered patients really have, and how much say medical experts have in choosing and coordinating patient care. Unless this paradoxical positioning of the key players in the health care debate is rectified, there is limited room for improvement.

Questions

1. The story of the first patient (with severe psoriasis) addresses the requirement for patients to fail therapy before insurance companies will reimburse advanced care. Why would insurance companies take this stance?

2. Examine the case of the patient who is concerned about losing disability benefits during recovery. If you were designing a health care system, how should "the point of recovery" be determined?

3. Is it possible for a system to both incentivize wellness and provide appropriate assistance for those with chronic illnesses?

4. How might you manage situations like these when you're in practice? How will you cope with possible feelings of helplessness as a caregiver when faced with such systemic obstacles?

—Sanjay Salgado

A Lack of Care: Why Medical Students Should Focus on Ferguson

December 2, 2014

Jennifer Tsai
Warren Alpert Medical School of Brown University
Class of 2017

YOU CAN'T ASK YOUR co-worker for narcotics the same way you can ask for extra Advil stashed in their purse or backpack. There are good reasons for this. Drugs like Advil or Tylenol carry little association with danger and can be easily bought at any local drugstore. While they are perfectly good for minimal pain relief from headaches or muscle soreness, they are underequipped for addressing major sources of pain. In comparison, opioid narcotics are serious painkillers. They carry risk of addiction and overdose, and can only be accessed with a physician prescription.

Now imagine you break your arm or leg, and the doctor in the emergency room prescribes you Tylenol.

To be clear, long bone fractures are often used in scientific studies specifically because they are always excruciating, and there is little range in the variation of patient pain. Breaking your leg or your arm hurts a lot, no matter how it happened.

Now if that broken bone is beneath black skin, the attending physician doing your initial work up and admittance exam is twice as likely to prescribe Tylenol for your fractured leg, and is twice as likely to prescribe opioid painkillers for the broken leg of the white patient next to you. In fact, in comparison to a white patient, a black one is half as likely to receive any sort of pain medication during an emergency room assessment of a broken bone.[1]

These statistics are not rare. African-American children are more likely than white children to be suspended from school or diagnosed with vague, psycho-behavioral ailments such as "oppositional defiance disorder."[2] Antipsychotic drugs, as opposed to counseling or therapy that look into child behavior as a fixable issue rather than a pathology, are prescribed four times more often to children covered by Medicaid as to children covered by private insurance.[3] This issue of class intersects with race and disproportionately impacts children of color. Black and Hispanic patients are less likely to be prescribed opioid pain medications that carry higher risk of abuse, trafficking and addiction.[4]

Pain and mental illness especially cannot be measured by pricking your finger or stepping on a scale. In the absence of quantitative measures, it is ultimately physician judgment that will determine how to treat a patient. Physicians, however, do not render their perceptions within a vacuum. The cultural makeup of America inevitably shapes physician perception of patient moral and social character, which is not unrelated to the doctor's formulation and judgment of that patient's medical issues.

These same perceptions of moral and social character explain why black men are more likely to be jailed for drug charges that white men more frequently commit, why in 2014 more than 80 percent of New York City stop-and-frisk suspects were people of color despite their constituting less than 30 percent of the local population, and why a young unarmed man can be shot in the middle of the street and left there for hours.[5,6]

The August 9, 2014 shooting of 18-year-old Michael Brown in Ferguson, Missouri is a recent and tangible illustration of how systemic racism operates and impacts the perception and treatment of black bodies. Although Michael Brown's death is generally understood as a political issue, it also illuminates current conditions of health care inequality. While issues of medicine and politics are often cast as different and discrete social and scientific realms, analysis of health care demonstrates that medicine is, at its heart, also a political issue. Indeed, the events that have unfolded in Ferguson have everything to do with why people of color in this country lose their health and lives at staggeringly higher rates in comparison to their white counterparts. Health care inequality cannot be understood outside the context of systemic racism. The understanding of Michael Brown's death as a function of institutional oppression helps to explain why individuals proclaiming an interest in medicine or health care disparities should have their attention focused on Ferguson. While the landscape regarding Ferguson is heavily dotted with scholars, civil rights leaders, politicians and journalists, attention from health care providers has remained largely absent. Just as the shooting of Michael Brown has helped the larger public recognize how the United States criminal justice system is racially biased, analyzing the event's foundations in institutional racism invites parallel scrutiny of our health care system. These same racial factors explain why both the American criminal justice system and the American health care system continue to produce extremely racialized outcomes despite both being supposedly and superficially race neutral. Our institutions are susceptible to the same vulnerabilities.

Ferguson helps us understand the racial climate that allows injustices to exist under seemingly race-blind policies. It is impossible to imagine a situation in which an unarmed white woman raising her hands in surrender would be shot by a police officer multiple times. This simple acknowl-edgment begs a number of questions about the structural forces that equate black individuals with criminals. Michael Brown, as an unarmed individual standing several feet away from pursuing officer Darren Wilson, could not have been seen as a threat in any instance except one where his identity as a black male had been previously framed as an inherent menace. Why are criminals so often imagined to be black men, and how does this conception create conditions in which unarmed black men can be shot on the street? Systemic racism is at the foundation of the forces that package and stereo-type young black men, that turn "blackness" into a pathology, and overall so greatly impact our systems' abilities to care for, adjudicate, and see popula-tions of color.

Michael Brown's body was attacked in the abstract before he was shot, it was attacked physically on the afternoon of August 9, and it continued to be attacked in the days and weeks following. In the days after the shooting, Bill Maher dubbed Brown a "thug" and a "criminal," while *The New York Times* suggested he was "no angel." Multiple media news outlets mobilized classic black tropes and labeled Brown as a "gang member," a "hulking thug" and a "ghetto rapper" with no consideration of why such descriptions, true or false, were relevant to the events surrounding his death. The controver-sy surrounding Michael Brown's character is further evidence of a system that unjustly scrutinizes certain identities. The injustice in question was an unlawful shooting situated in a culture of police brutality, and yet pub-lic conversation often involves Brown's history as if it could justify Darren Wilson's actions, as if a supposedly moral evaluation can validate a legal one. These perceptions of Michael Brown demonstrate the kind of value judgments and stereotypes structural racism continues to foster. There are thousands of 18-year-olds of every race who smoke, rap and drink, and yet it is so much more often young men of color that are presupposed as "thugs" and threats to society.

The cultural biases that led Officer Wilson to shoot Brown permeate our culture, and this culture does not cease to exist within medical schools and inside hospital wards. Inevitably, these biases influence the conditions in which doctors shape their decisions regarding diagnostic recommendation, treatment prescription, and patient understanding. Essentialism, the over-simplified assumption or perception that certain populations have congru-ent values, behaviors, or tendencies, is a major operation, contribution, and byproduct of racism. Essentializing young black men, and indeed any and all populations, creates barriers to equal care and access by influencing the way doctors understand, listen, see, and treat their patients.

This manifestation of institutional oppression folds directly into racial profiling. Black patients are still associated with sickle cell anemia despite evidence that shows rates of sickle cell increase in all geographic areas with high prevalence of malaria, including Greece, Turkey, and India.[7] Gay men are still prohibited from donating blood because of a historical association with HIV and AIDS. Asian women are still targeted in abortion clinics because of presumptions regarding cultural infanticide. Assumptions of patient character or capability impact medical practice by casting patients in roles that doctors expect them to fill. Systemic racism explains why doctors may assume black patients are more likely to exhibit drug-seeking behavior and exaggerate their pain. It explains why physicians may unconsciously presuppose black patients to be too irresponsible to self-administer addictive opioid drug treatments, have higher predisposition towards substance abuse, or require antipsychotic medication. It explains why we cannot create solutions to health care disparities without recognizing the ways in which systemic racism prevents equal quality and access to health. The prejudices on display in Ferguson can just as readily be found in the waiting room.

At the center of this issue is a startling fact: if the life expectancy of African Americans in the United States equaled that of their white counterparts, there would be 83,750 fewer black deaths a year.[8] In certain cities, one out of three black deaths would not have occurred if black and white mortality rates were the same. Black infant mortality is two-and-a-half times higher than it is for whites.[9] Black patients are less likely to be put on transplant lists, receive aggressive cardiovascular intervention, and receive hip fracture repair; yet they are more likely to receive lower limb amputation as result of delayed care.[10,11,12] The statistics are as jarring as they are extensive. Again and again, studies show that even when controlling for income, occupation and education, African-American citizens receive lower quality care.

To me, this circles back to issues of medical education. While medical knowledge is heavily rooted in the biomedical model, the provision of health care needs to explicitly address the social context of medicine. It is not productive to be "race-blind" in a racist society, and we need to directly address issues of race within health care if we want to make progress. For those interested in health care disparities, the events in Ferguson should not be seen as a peripheral current events issue, but rather an increasingly important platform by which we can better understand how and why racial inequalities continue to exist. The shooting of Michael Brown remains a primary access point in assessing how racism dictates not only racialized health outcomes and access to care, but also one's ability to receive equal treatment and quality of care in the context of personal, and thus physician, bias. Questions about health care access, policy, insurance and care quality are very much discussions of human rights, dignity and citizenship.

Health care professionals need to be more critical of the ways in which individual perceptions shaped by systemic racism often leak into practice. The unconscious formation of these stereotypes is dangerous because they often remain unacknowledged and are thus extra insidious by virtue of their subtlety. The doctors prescribing Advil to black patients in lieu of the opioid painkillers they are more apt to give their white patients are likely not trying to discriminate — their decisions may be imperceptibly influenced by inclinations they cannot name or identify succinctly. Similarly, Darren Wilson perhaps did not make the conscious decision to attack Brown in a way he would not have pursued a white individual, but he learned and lived in a society in which being black divorces one from "angelic" qualities and can apparently warrant suspicion and six bullet holes. These issues do not revolve around the isolated mistakes of individual doctors or policemen, but rather systems that are structurally unsound. It is not a question about bad apples, but tainted soil. Implicit biases exist even in people, and doctors, who are vigorously anti-racist. Understanding the legacy of systemic racism helps us to recognize the ways we ourselves may be complicit in structural racism by virtue of acting within a system that is structurally designed to give lower quality health care to the people who are most disempowered and marginalized. At the end of the day, while recognizing institutional forces can help explain widespread inequality, institutions are run by people, and until we allocate greater responsibility and accountability to the people who perpetuate this issue, this problem will never be solved.

Michael Brown's death is one symptom of the sickness systemic racism produces. Like symptoms, it decries a larger problem and prompts us to search for its root cause, and the breadth of its infection. The public often extrapolates that medicine, as an extension of science, is an objective, factual practice. Even as medical students, we learn in our textbooks the histological characteristics of cells, the mechanisms of glomerular filtration, pulmonary measurements, biochemical pathways and diagnostic tests used to identify symptoms and syndromes. It is easy to presume that medicine is colorblind, and the care we give a rational process. But cells are not people, and science is not health care. Doctoring is an inherently social discipline that revolves around patient-doctor interaction, and the few minutes doctors have with their patients last only long enough to develop snapshot judgments that go on to dictate the diagnosis and care patients will receive. Pretending medicine is a rational exercise denies its role as a social force and allows its continued participation in structural racism to go undiagnosed.

On a case-to-case basis, in which structural racism manifests as higher rates of amputation, fewer follow-ups, less effective pain medication, or preconceived assumptions of ability, it may be easy to assume that the racism that creates health care disparities is not quite as insidious as the police brutality we see splashed across our newspapers and TV screens. The diminished scrutiny the medical system receives by virtue of its reputation as an objective practice, however, makes it harder to see that health care itself is also a primary source and outlet of institutional racism. Michael Brown is one of many victims systemic racism has claimed, and until doctors acknowledge the position of medicine within institutional racism, our health care system will continue to reproduce tragedies like Ferguson, even in the absence of a smoking gun.

Questions

1. Should medical students focus on Ferguson?

2. Do you feel your medical education has provided sufficient training in caring for patients from different racial, ethnic and cultural backgrounds? If not, what can be improved in your training?

3. Discuss curriculum changes you would like to see at your institution in regards to racial and other disparities in health care.

4. What instances have you witnessed during your medical training in which "health care itself is also a primary source and outlet of institutional racism?"

—Aleena Paul

Physicians-in-Transit:
The Blizzard of 2015

January 30, 2015

Jacob Walker
Boston University School of Medicine
Class of 2016

A WINTER CHILL CAN TRIGGER quite the flurry of activity on the floors of an urban safety-net hospital. Patients trail in from the cold with a telling set of problems: their asthma seems to be getting worse; shoveling caused a worrying chest pain; their toes are changing color; they have nowhere else to go. Senior staff begin wandering the wards, desperate to create room for those in need. It becomes a hospital-wide effort to get healthy bodies out the door in order to make way for an influx of the sick. And on one such January morning, the solution for an overflowing and quickly growing roster of the sick and weary was just a single step: hand out taxi vouchers and the beds will empty.

—

I want you to pause and think critically about how you get to and from work every day. How long does it take? How much walking does it require? What modes of transportation do you use? Is it expensive? Do you know how you would get to work on crutches? In a wheelchair? How about in a snowstorm? Or without a driver's license?

I ask because I have the unheard-of luxury of writing this from home on a dangerously snowy weekday afternoon. That's because like the majority of health care workers in Boston, I rely on public transportation to get to work and any major weather calamity that disrupts public transit massively disrupts the entire city's health care network. Hospitals cancelled surgeries, closed clinics and provided makeshift sleeping quarters for staff. Local journalist Martha Bebinger on WBUR commented that all but one of the city's 73 community health centers were forced to close, largely because of the inability to get staff to where they needed to be.[1]

But these are extraordinary circumstances. It's not every day that Rhode Island needs to clarify their "health care worker emergency transportation process" or a Framingham hospital needs to house more than 30 extra staff overnight.[2] And this mess of a travel situation gave me pause to consider the surprisingly complex process patients need to face on a *normal* day every time they visit their doctor.

—

That the solution to a precariously overcrowded hospital is to provide *taxi vouchers* makes a great deal of sense when considering the often-overlooked challenge of physically moving people about a city. What better way to get stable yet frail and tired patients home than to conveniently *chauffeur* them home? It's an aspect of care from which most medical staff are often removed. Our patients come to us either by their own accord or by ambulance. We don't need to guide them to our clinics; they simply appear there. Most of the transportation management that needs to occur happens outside of the exam room. Support staff are usually the ones coordinating ambulance rides, wheelchair-accessible vans, handicap license plates, or parking vouchers. But not every patient will know that these services are available and often the issue of "how do you get to your appointments?" falls through the cracks.

Anecdotally, I have had a patient spend an extra night in the hospital because a wheelchair-friendly ride was not available. I have had patients leave appointments in a rush because the meter was running or miss appointments all together because they could not find a parking spot or the rain kept them from waiting for the bus. We can assess these barriers subjectively as well.[3] We know that transportation is a major hurdle for patients needing procedures like colonoscopies and outpatient surgeries, as well as to follow-up on essential exams such as an abnormal Pap smear.[4,5,6] It is critical to account for and address these physical obstacles because even as we hurdle towards the age of telemedicine (while simultaneously reviving the routine of in-home visits) we will still, on occasion, need to get patients to a clinic. It remains an unfortunate reality that physicians can't stop the rains or become the masters of urban planning needed to fix "the parking situation," but we can remember to ask our patients some critical questions that apply just as aptly to getting around town as to coping with illness:

Where are you going? And how can I help?

Questions

1. A blizzard ... a flat tire ... a traffic jam. Each of us has experienced difficulty getting to work. When was the last time you had such an experience? What were your feelings in the midst of the calamity?

2. Now think of your patients, and your patience when the clinic schedule shows '15 minutes late' on the screen. Where is that line between what is acceptable for us as medical professionals and what is acceptable for each of our patients?

3. In medical school, we learn about patient-centered care. Is there such an entity as "physician-centered care," in which the health care system emphasizes physician convenience over patient convenience? Is this ever an acceptable way to deliver health care? Why or why not?

4. For a moment, be an exceptional mind at the Google team. What is one thing you could create or change that would make transportation for our patients a simpler affair?

—Brent Bjornsen

My Black Eyes

March 11, 2015

Jessica Ubanyionwu
University of Texas Medical Branch at Galveston
Class of 2017

L OOKING OUT AND SEEING the beautiful colors that surround me, I always used to feel bad for those not able to experience the power of the colors of the world. See, I was born without sight. No ability to distinguish red from white. For the longest time I thought I had missed out on something and I was mad at my creator for not giving me such a blessing.

As I walk around my medical school campus, I embrace the blessing that was given to me to be able to see. I never knew that one day I would get to see the color that was associated with the touch. Black was no longer the only color I knew. There were so many shades of color and they all mattered.

But in that ability to see, came more than what I had bargained for.

My name is Jessica. No nicknames. It was the name that I had identified myself with all my life. I was smart; well, at least that is what people told me. I made good grades and I tried to be a leader in everything I did. I felt like I worked for everything I had received, and I was going to be a doctor.

Affirmative action. Diversity. A destined amount of black people per class.

"How did you get in? Are you the nurse? You want to be a doctor? Why?"

I had never in my life felt that I was less than the expectation. These people did not know me, but their opinion about me was permanent. I had no say as to what they were going to think of me and it did not matter what I did because I lived in a body that had a prejudged color. The feeling grew in me that people thought I had made it this far because I was African-American. Because they needed a certain amount of blacks per class to meet some type of quota. I no longer earned it. I did not work hard to get into medical school; it was given to me.

Maybe everyone should experience not being able to see. That feeling of appreciating the world with four senses. Recognizing that color is supposed to be beautiful. It shouldn't tailor your heart in a way that alters the mindset of people walking in a different shadow than yourself.

I've learned to accept the fact that it is hard to change the opinions of others. I have accepted the fact that people are going to think less of me even after I prove otherwise. I have accepted the fact that this is the world I live in. But I have not accepted that this is permanent.

I wish the world were colorblind.

Questions

1. How do our cultural backgrounds color the way in which we view medicine and medical education?

2. What steps can you take as a future health professional to increase the presence of members of underrepresented groups in medicine?

3. What does it mean to have "diverse" medical profession? Is it an important concept to try and achieve? Why or why not?

—Aleena Paul

Mine

March 13, 2015

Damien Zreibe
University of South Florida Morsani College of Medicine
Class of 2018

You claim that *my* choice breaks *your* heart,
as if mine isn't shattered and cracked.
You think I don't know how beautiful he'd be,
or wonder how he'd walk, talk and act.

You think that I'm evil and going to hell,
but my beliefs do not equal yours.
You yell in my face and protest my right,
— starting fights, starting chaos, and wars.

You claim that you know my story,
that I chose death and that I'm out of line.
Little do you see, that I did choose life;
but the life that I chose, was mine.

Author's note: This is a poem from the perspective of a woman who had an abortion, inspired by a passion for the right of a patient to choose freely.

Questions

1. What does it mean to have "a choice?" What are the choices that are being made in the span of this poem?

2. What responsibility do physicians have to provide a service that they do not believe in personally or morally? What if a physician was the only one in the area able to provide this service in a safe manner?

3. Who has the power in society to make choices? How can the ability to make choices be taken away from a person?

—Aleena Paul

On Silence:
The Limits of Professionalism
April 7, 2015

Jennifer Hong
Emory School of Medicine
Class of 2018

I N HER MEMOIR "The Cancer Journals," radical feminist and civil rights
activist Audre Lorde documented her experiences as a woman with breast
cancer recovering from a mastectomy. Lorde was a black lesbian and patient who is "defined as *other* in every group I am a part of. I'm the outsider,
both strength and weakness."[1]

An individual who identified as a minority on multiple levels, Lorde
used her memoir as a platform to voice her experiences as a marginalized
woman of color and patient in a patriarchal, white supremacist medical
system and society. She was a "post-mastectomy woman who believes our
feelings need voice in order to be recognized, respected, and of use." In the
memoir and throughout her life, Lorde articulated the relationship between
voice and power, how the command of a language and the ability to vocalize
those commands are assertions of power.

The ability to speak manifests as the ability to communicate our wishes
and desires effectively. This theme is much easier to identify in books, with
obvious buzzwords like "interrupt" or "drowned out," but it is not a nebu-
lous concept that only exists in fiction. Instead, this relationship reflects the
social dynamics of reality. Studies have shown that the right to speak is "intimately tied with rights to power," with a quantitative measure of asserting
power through speech being the number of unilateral changes in conversation.[2] The literal interruptions that occur in daily conversations are therefore common real manifestations of power dynamics embodied by voice.

Thus, this power is not necessarily singular — one can speak but not
be heard or be overridden, thus effectively being silenced. This ability to
silence, therefore, is one that belongs to the individual or collective group in
power. Those that remain in power in society are the ones with the ability to
speak *and* be heard, who also hold the ability to dismiss the voices of others.

The relationship between voice and power can easily be seen in our medical education as we learn the vital skill of building rapport with patients. We are cautioned to avoid over-speaking: let silence linger, giving patients the opportunity to speak. Before the migration to patient-centered care, doctors' conversations with patients were (and may still be) largely one-sided: the doctor is the speaker, while the patient is the recipient. By teaching us to "let silence linger" and encouraging us to listen to patients' stories, medical education is shifting the power dynamic from one of explicit hierarchy to one of collaboration — hence, patient-centered care.

Silence is an important tool that physicians need to learn how to use. The patient-physician relationship is a strange, special one because the physician is privy to so much of the patients' personal lives. Given the physician's historical power, physicians are in a much greater position to do harm to the patient than vice versa. As such, it is important to remain silent when the patient is speaking; after all, it is not the provider's place to judge the patient's actions because judgment contributes nothing positive to the relationship.

But while medical school teaches us how to use silence as a method of building better patient relationships for our future practices, it also grooms us to use silence as a protective mechanism. Instead of silence for the patients, the emphasis of silence is often placed in the context of professionalism and therefore silence on behalf of the medical sphere. As medical students, we reflect both our respective institutions as well as the larger community of medical professionals. Regardless of collaboration, our white coats are still a huge status symbol and as the wearers, we need to be particularly careful with what we say.

The ultimate rule for a physician is the Hippocratic Oath: "Do no harm." This oath is mostly interpreted in the explicit manner of doing no physical harm, but also encompasses other forms of harm as well: mental, social and so forth. To avoid doing these less tangible forms of harm, we believe that the trick is often to simply be silent and consequently neutral. In this narrow reading of the Hippocratic Oath, by expressing no opinion, especially one that would clash with the patient's own, we believe we do no harm and abide by the physicians' role of ultimately treating the patient and nothing else.

As such, we are taught that medicine is supposed to be an "apolitical" sphere — the relevant facts are overwhelmingly medical, and any mention of social factors like race are instead framed as genetic. To mention race and its non-medical implications — namely, racism — is seen as irrelevant to the medicine. Multiple times, I have heard from medical students that racism and sexism are not related to medicine and public health. Additionally, these topics are sticky and dangerous — after all, to many, racism is "over" because we live in a "post-racial" society of supposed equal opportunity.

Between the doctor and patient, silence should be extended to allow room for the patient's voice. But what about silence in response to factors affecting patients that aren't necessarily medically related — topics that are awkward, uncomfortable, and require acknowledgment of privilege both in and outside of medicine? Silence is therefore multifaceted: it can be enforced in a top-down, oppressive manner, and it can be allowed, a willing collaboration. The two, however, can be misconstrued as being identical.

Last month, I went to a talk given by acclaimed author Salman Rushdie. The topic was on the pursuit of liberty and how freedom of speech needs to be protected, as our fundamental rights to liberty are being slowly stripped away by the current age of "political corrected-ness." To be funny takes courage now, Rushdie said, citing the Charlie Hebdo attacks and the response to Seth Rogen and James Franco's "The Interview." By Rushdie's argument, we are so bound by political "corrected-ness" and its repercussions that we are silenced from truly speaking what we think.

To be frank, I disagree. We — in medicine and in society as a whole — are not silenced by "political corrected-ness." There is a significant difference between being unable to make jokes at the expense of marginalized individuals due to "political corrected-ness" and being unable to speak out against the systems marginalizing these individuals in the first place by being silenced or dismissed. The attacks on Charlie Hebdo were condemned internationally as acts of terrorism and violence, and rightfully so. However, there was not quite the same kind of unanimous condemnation for the acts of terrorism and violence against Muslims displayed in the movie "American Sniper," acts that continue in reality to this day. There was not condemnation for two white men deciding that they could belittle the sufferings of North Koreans by making "The Interview" into a comedy. Instead, these movies are heralded as patriotic: staunch defendants of freedom of speech and the embodiment of true Americans. In fact, many have used freedom of speech to defend the recent SAE fraternity members' absolutely blatant racism and condemn their expulsion — after all, how can we punish freedom of speech when it so embodies all America represents, when we all have a right to be intolerant?[3]

Thus, silence and voice work in different ways for different people. There are existing systems in place that favor certain groups over others — in other words, being able to speak and be heard, as well as the ability to silence, belongs to individuals who are privileged. Being white grants privilege. Being male grants privilege. And ultimately, being a physician grants privilege.

We have the power to speak over patients, plain and simple, but we shouldn't. If we are truly patient advocates, we need to know when to be silent and when to be vocal. When with the patient, either in the clinic office or at the bedside, silence can be a powerful tool that we employ on our own behalf so that we can learn what the patient needs. But when outside of the direct patient interaction, we as physicians shouldn't be silent. Rather, we need to be conscious of the privilege afforded to us as physicians and recognize that our voices have power to change the existing racist and classist systems that continue to devalue the lives of minorities, inside and outside of our practice.

Advocacy, therefore, is not confined to the clinic. As physicians, we should not simply be "apolitical" when it comes to matters outside of medicine, because factors outside medicine affect not just our patients but our practice and our society as a whole. Essentially, we cannot *afford* to be apolitical and focus "just on the science" because that is a luxury that others do not have.

To be silent in the face of systematic injustices — legislative, medical, social and otherwise — is to be complicit in them. To believe that medicine is an insular, neutral field is naïve. Access to care is tied to socioeconomic class. Socioeconomic class is tied to race. And race has always been and still is tied to vastly varying levels of privilege and opportunities. To assume that a patient can simply abide by medical suggestions without any context for their social situation is to ignore a historical system of oppression that extends to multiple spheres, of which medicine is only one. How and why do geographical food deserts predominately affect lower socioeconomic communities? How do legislative barriers to reproductive health disproportionately target women in poverty and why are those women overwhelmingly black or brown? How does being constantly exposed to racism contribute to the prevalence of hypertension among the black American community? If we ignore these questions and deem them to be unrelated to medicine, then we are ignoring huge factors that perpetuate the injustices that continue to oppress entire communities.

Ultimately, what I want to point out is that silence is not always neutral. On the contrary, silence is often a sign of complicity, and the protective silence that the medical community often employs can and does do harm. Contrary to what we may believe, in most cases, silence is not apolitical; silence in the face of great injustices done to others is either willful ignorance of the injustice or full acknowledgment of the injustice's existence without acknowledging its nature.

The natural course of this conversation turns to that of race and the ongoing events of systematic violence against minorities in the United States, particularly against black and Muslim lives. In the wake of the non-indictments of Michael Brown and Eric Garner's killers, there was national movement from the medical student community to protest the threat to black lives. This movement stemmed from students who felt that a great injustice had been committed not just against the individuals involved, but against the entire black community in the United States. This movement stemmed from students who felt that they still face systematic injustices to this day, and that silence could no longer be tolerated, as continued silence was the same as effectively ignoring the problem.

Here, silent professionalism reaches its limits. Being a professional does not mean not having opinions. It means not having opinions that continue to marginalize individuals who are already disadvantaged. Being a professional does not mean not rocking the boat or not tackling the status quo when the status quo perpetually favors one group of individuals over another. Though it is understandably easier to focus on the medicine because that's what we're taught and hired to do, ignoring the injustices both within and outside of medicine does violate the Hippocratic Oath, because silence — real, nearly tangible, oppressive weight — can and does do harm.

Questions

1. Do you agree with the author's statements that "silence is a sign of complicity?" Why or why not?

2. Reflect on situations where medical professionals' silence has done damage either to patients or to the profession itself.

3. Do you believe physicians should take a greater role in politics?

4. What is your reaction to physicians who have become "celebrities" and who make statements that contradict the stances held by the majority of the profession?

—Aleena Paul

My White Coat Costume

April 8, 2015

Jes Minor
Yale School of Medicine
Class of 2022

O N THE DAY OF MY white coat ceremony, I felt like a pretender. I squirmed in the rigid, wooden seat, staring at the gilded columns and towering proscenium of the hall, wondering when I'd be found out. I imagined them calling me to the stage, slipping on the coat, then seeing me in it and saying, "Well, that doesn't look quite right."

I must have worn my thoughts like a billboard on my forehead, because the dean read my mind. "I'm sure you're all feeling a bit of 'impostor-syndrome' right now," he said, "but trust me, admissions doesn't make mistakes."

Maybe I'm not alone, I thought.

When the speaker, Dr. Miller, rose to the stage, he began talking about the meaning of the white coat. I felt excited: whether I deserved it or not, I would soon wear that coat like a stamp of approval on my dreams.

Dr. Miller told a story of a patient he'd never met, but who had recognized Dr. Miller in the hospital as a physician.

"When I asked him why," Dr. Miller continued, "he told me, 'You just look like how a doctor should look.'"

I squinted at him. I tried to see what that patient had seen. Behind the podium, I saw an older, white man with pink cheeks, glasses, a tie, and yes, a white coat. I scanned the stage and saw several of his lookalikes: all white, almost all men, as though the feature figures of so many Norman Rockwell paintings had come together to celebrate how good and 'doctorly' they looked.

Not one of them looked like *me*. Me, with the dark curly hair, the deep olive skin, and the high cheekbones that hint at my distant indigenous ancestry.

I knew then that my instincts had been correct: that I didn't fit the mold of a Yale-educated doctor. That knowledge steeled my resolve to prove them wrong.

I rose to the stage and reached my arms into the white sleeves my professor held behind me. I decided then to think of my white coat as a prop in a costume box: when I wore it, I would transform myself into someone fantastic, like a doctor, and no one would question me. My childhood beliefs on dress-up made it simple: glitter dress plus tiara equals princess, so white coat plus stethoscope equals doctor. I looked forward to playing that part.

After the ceremony, I slapped on an extrovert's smile and dove headfirst into medical school. I began to feel different from my classmates early on in orientation.

"Where are you from?" they would ask, one or two questions into the conversation.

"New Jersey," I would answer, pressing the edges of my spurious smile. They would nod and emit a bemused "oh."

"I thought you looked more ethnic," one said.

More ethnic, I mused. The term prompted me to wonder how much of my heritage could be read in my skin.

As I sat with these classmates in lecture, a parade of white men imbued me with knowledge of signaling pathways and cranial nerves, but my professionalism instructor couldn't distinguish between "ethnicity" and "race." That lecture on health disparities faltered at the sound of his uncertain fingers scratching the stifled skin under his collar.

Later in the anatomy lab, our surgeon preceptors sidled up to the one man in my group and guided his hands through the most complicated techniques. I, and the two other women on my dissection team, craned over their shoulders, trying to broach this forbidden space where male surgeons primed their kind for prestige.

Worst of all, despite my white coat costume, my patients saw through me.

"Let's talk about the difficulty breathing," I began, practicing the phrases I learned in class. "Start with how it began and walk me through today." Our patient looked up from her bed, right over my five-feet and one inch, and spoke directly to the white man in my group. I plucked the hangnails on my fingers as I nodded along to her story.

Before coming to medical school, I was hopeful. I believed that my understanding of color discrimination, of privilege and power dynamics, and of gender and sexual diversity would allow me to treat patients with greater sensitivity. I felt confident that my scholarly framework for social inequities would enable me to combat them. I trusted that my words, so saturated with compassion, were enough to forge bonds with the people I'd serve. I had not anticipated that I would become the object of my own inquiries on social justice: that my gender expression, my size, and my skin color would be the variables I'd study in evaluating my shortcomings as a developing physician.

I'll be a doctor someday, but I might not be the kind that the patient in

Dr. Miller's story expected. I've learned that some of us — those with deeper complexions, short stature or unmasculine bodies — might be destined to pretend. So, I'll put on my white coat and put on a good show. I will make-believe enough to make my patients believe in me.

Questions

1. What aspects of you and your background might keep you from feeling that you belong in your white coat?

2. What pressures are there to conform to a specific image of professionalism in medicine? Who decides what is "doctorly" enough, and should this image be changed?

3. We receive a lot of training in how to treat our patients. How can we be better prepared for how our patients will treat us, based on their own prejudices and past experiences?

—Tolulope Omojokun

Street Medicine

April 21, 2015

Ajay Koti
University of South Florida Morsani College of Medicine
Class of 2017

A TORRENTIAL THUNDERSTORM forced nearly the entire homeless population of Tampa Heights out from under their tents and awnings in favor of the more generous cover of a highway overpass. It was the closest Tampa had come to a publicly funded homeless shelter.

"And I was running, you know, just — getting out — just goin', man." An older veteran named Detroit closed his eyes and reminisced. He twisted his trunk — "*swoosh, swish*," running from the sound of gunfire in his memory. "And then, *BAM!*" He clapped his hands and the sound reverberated through the rain and interstate traffic. He outlined a spot on his jeans where a bullet tore through his thigh a quarter-century ago. Detroit had to spend several months in a VA hospital recovering from the wound. He had incurred the injury not through combat, but as a direct consequence of his homelessness; he suffered from being in "the wrong place at the wrong time."

Around when Detroit was relearning to walk, Dr. Jim Withers was taking his first steps through Pittsburgh. Soon after arriving, he launched Operation Safety Net: a street medicine program and approach to health care that has inspired hundreds of medical students and physicians across the country. Today, there are roughly 40 street medicine programs all over the globe, including the one in Tampa.

William, a wiry man in a stained green sweater, was another member of the homeless community finding shelter under the highway. He was drenched from the rain and had no medical concerns, only romantic ones. "I've had some relationship problems," he said sheepishly. I contemplated changing the subject — I felt even less qualified to weigh in on relationship issues than on medical issues — but Will was persistent. To my surprise, he pointed to a woman sitting on the curb a few yards away. "She really helped me out, man, when I got into town, getting clothes and shit. And I wanted to try and work it out with her, but she just wasn't interested ... But I really like her..." This wasn't the story of some past relationship gone sour — this was an ongoing, active situation that started on the streets. I waited to hear more, but before Will could continue, Detroit approached and asked me to take a look at his ankle.

Will hovered nearby, patiently waiting as Detroit hobbled to the curb and gingerly removed his sneaker. A large callus had formed over his right Achilles tendon, the product of a nasty cut and poorly fitting shoes. I fumbled for my penlight; Detroit produced a pocket flashlight of his own, peering intently as I smeared iodine on the exposed ankle. In hushed tones, he delved into the story about the gunshot wound he suffered on the streets of the city that became his namesake.

"I really wish I had a better pair of shoes for you," I said, looking up from the foot. Detroit chuckled at my suggestion. A bandage, a fresh pair of socks, a fist bump, and he limped back into the rain.

A police cruiser rolled through the underpass. "Fuckin' PD," Will said. "They probably want to harass people, always fucking telling folks to move along."

"Move along where?"

Will laughed. "Fuck, man, they don't give a shit."

Cities across the state of Florida have become notorious for policies banning public eating, sleeping and displays of personal property. Ninety-year-old chef Arnold Abbott made headlines when he was arrested in Fort Lauderdale for serving dinner to homeless individuals. To its credit, Tampa does not enforce anti-homeless ordinances with quite as much zeal, but the anti-homeless attitudes stubbornly remain.

As the downpour eased, the scores of people under the overpass began to disperse.

"You guys have to do essays, papers, shit like that?" Will asked. "Write about this. Write about us."

Questions

1. What barriers impede health care for homeless persons?

2. What are your personal biases? What biases have you witnessed toward homeless persons seeking care in the emergency room?

3. What other populations do you feel have stories that medical students could benefit from hearing, but so often go untold?

—Natalie Wilcox

Our Patients

The Chair

October 6, 2012

Ben Ferguson
University of Chicago Pritzker School of Medicine
Class of 2013

A LITTLE HUMOR GOES A long way with a lot of patients. The degree to which a positive attitude — on their part and ours — can help them get through a difficult time in their lives never ceases to amaze me. One patient came to us with massive lower extremity swelling and an ejection fraction of 15 percent. He was an inpatient for over a month and had a Foley catheter for more than three weeks. He had an indwelling peritoneal catheter to drain the massive buildup of ascitic fluid at regular intervals. He sat upright in a chair for the majority of this time, not able to walk or even stand because of his heart function and his trunks for legs. He slept in the chair. He ate in the chair. He urinated from the chair. He awaited evaluation for surgical candidacy in the chair. He hated the chair.

Yet, every morning, he would have a new quip, a new off-color shot at the consulting services, a new joke, a new self-deprecating observation that would have us in stitches. He ripped on the chair. He made jokes about the chair's mama. He made me laugh more than any patient I've encountered, and I made him laugh too. (I almost made him desaturate once or twice too, but it was worth it. He told me so once he caught his breath.) He demonstrated to us that it's possible to stay positive in such dire straits, and it's possible to emotionally thrive. He showed that making light of a tough situation is not somewhere within denial, but somewhere well beyond acceptance.

Bringing a little personality to this method adds a certain human quality, a particular realism that categorical, tenuous professionalism never could. The patient later died waiting for a heart. But he was sharp, he was happy, and he was rid of the chair.

Questions

1. Do you agree with the author's statement that being able to laugh at a situation is indicative of a patient's acceptance of his or her circumstances? Why or why not?

2. Is it ever acceptable of a physician to make light of or joke about a patient's condition? In what situations might this be appropriate?

—Theresa Yang

My Contribution

November 19, 2012

Kerri Vincenti
George Washington University School of Medicine
Class of 2014

N OT EVERYONE HAS THE pleasure, or should I say honor, of being a part
of the miracle that is life; even fewer get to say that they witness and influence that miracle every day. As a medical student, I have been privy to a
whole new world of opportunities that have opened my eyes to how fragile
life truly is and how much of a difference one person can make to affect
the life (or death) of another. What's more, at some point in this journey, I
became strikingly aware of the fact that at every level of medical training,
there is an air of responsibility — a feeling mixed with both uneasiness and
pride — that drives doctors, nurses and other medical professionals alike,
to contribute what they can for the benefit of their patient's health. At the
height of this realization, I found myself wondering what I could contribute
to those I serve with such little experience and knowledge.

It was the beginning of my third year of medical school — a time when
I felt like I was being flung into the fire of wards with no more armor than
the knowledge I had attained from my long-forgotten board review and an
eagerness to learn that was often shadowed by my transparent fear of being
wrong. I started my ward experience on internal medicine. It was a good
idea in theory; after all, I figured I would remember the most amount of
information based on the proximity to having just completed Step 1, and it
would provide a solid foundation for every other rotation to follow. I was
soon assigned my first patient, a complicated case of course, and like a
good third-year student, I looked up "pertinent" information with my newly purchased UpToDate subscription, discussed my proposed plan of care
with the intern, presented the differential on rounds to the attending, and
went home (exhausted) to make time to study some more. Days turned into
weeks for my patient, and I became increasingly frustrated that the team
(that I) couldn't figure out what was wrong. She was sick, partly from her

own doing, but regardless of why she was there, she needed our help and expected (rightfully so) that we would be able to "fix her."

About two weeks into the rotation, I pondered over the situation. I had seen many patients come and go from my care at that point, but the first patient was still in that same hospital bed I had found her in on my first day. I began visiting her more frequently in the afternoons, forgoing my usual time to do research. I didn't know if we were going to be able to help her given her frail state and the fact that we had exhausted several likely tests two to three times over, but I did know that she didn't have many visitors (none that I could recall, actually) so I figured she was probably lonely. At first, she met my kindness with bitterness and scorn, but day after day, my persistence slowly chipped away at her veil of anger to reveal a fearful but hopeful woman. I didn't have much to offer in terms of medical knowledge because I didn't fully understand half of what was going on myself. I couldn't even explain to her why she couldn't eat anything for the thousandth time because of some study she was going to get the next day (which I honestly couldn't explain very well, either). But I sat and listened. I listened to her talk about her new grand baby and how she wanted to see her for her birthday; I listened to her cry as she admitted that she didn't want to die and that she wasn't ready to let go of all the things she had left to do; I listened to her talk about God and how He had sent me to her so she could find the strength to change her ways once she got discharged.

The day finally came when she was going to go home (three days before my four week rotation was to end). I went in to check on her as usual in preparation for morning rounds, and despite my sheer exhaustion from having been on call the night before, the joy on her face made me smile uncontrollably. We'd finally gotten her condition under control. We hadn't really fixed her, but she was strong enough to leave, so it was time to say goodbye. Going into the rotation, I never would have guessed that one patient could teach me so much about how much I could contribute to her care, not by the disciplined application of new knowledge that I would learn, but by the unrestrained expression of the compassion that brought me to the field in the first place. As a student, it wasn't my "job" care to care about the disease — to know everything about it or to have all the answers for how to treat it (although I ultimately did have to learn these things). It was my duty and responsibility to care about the patient — to comfort, listen, and be present for her at a time in her life when she was most vulnerable — so she would know her well-being meant something to someone, even if that someone was just a third-year medical student.

Questions

1. How did the author make a "contribution" to the care for the patient despite her limited medical knowledge?

2. How should medical students deal with the frustration the author describes when faced with patients whose medical problems seem unsolvable?

3. Can you think of other scenarios in medicine in which compassion might be as, or perhaps more, useful than clinical intervention?

4. Do you believe that, as the author states, it wasn't her "job" to care about the disease? Why or why not?

—Angelica D'Aiello

Don't Judge a Book by Its Cover: A Complex Twist in a Patient with Diabetic Ketoacidosis

October 10, 2013

Manik Aggarwal
Texas A&M Health Science Center College of Medicine
Class of 2014

HERE WAS A 45-year-old Type 1 diabetic who presented to the emergency department in a near coma with diabetic ketoacidosis. The diagnosis seemed clear as day, with some of the classic presenting signs: polyuria, polydipsia, hyperglycemia, high anion gap, low serum bicarbonate and presence of ketones in the urine. She was admitted and treated appropriately. Once she was stabilized, the human interaction and history-taking began, which proved to be far more convoluted.

She thoroughly explained her history that started with a diabetes diagnosis in her early 20s. At that time, she presented to the emergency department with a bout of viral gastroenteritis that presumably triggered the initial episode of diabetic ketoacidosis.

Her social history was far more complex. She admitted to alcoholism reluctantly yet openly talked about her recent cocaine and methamphetamine abuse, and made a few subtle yet poignant remarks hinting towards domestic violence at home. She talked about a daughter that hated her, a mother that abandoned her, and a diagnosis that limited her. Although her immediate assessment and plan were straightforward and successful, something unexpected happened the following night.

Her sugars dropped to the mid-40s. She was immediately given orange juice and sugar tablets. She was stabilized and slept comfortably through the night. I saw her the following morning during breakfast and observed her enjoying her coffee with three sugar packets and her pancakes with molasses syrup.

This patient seemed to demonstrate an awareness of her condition and an avoidance of another hypoglycemic state. Perhaps our insulin regimen was aggressive — and likely too aggressive — for our medium-sized lady. The following day, her sugar began to creep into the 200s. Then we saw a

148

300, then a 400, then a 500. What were we doing or what was happening in her body to account for such dramatic changes in blood sugar? We weren't entirely sure, but were told by the patient that these fluctuations are consistent with her home readings. She said that she rarely goes down to the 70s and has adequate hypoglycemic awareness, but regularly yet inexplicably reaches the 500 mark on a weekly basis.

Her outpatient endocrinologist, who was not affiliated with our hospital, confirmed the story and told our team that this was a difficult-to-control Type 1 diabetic. He was certainly right; in a matter of 48 hours, her sugars had initially presented at 800, stabilized at 140, dropped to 70, went up to 500 and now had yet another episode of 80.

After a very eventful and painstaking week that involved additional sugar swings, patient-nurse and patient-physician confrontations and support from social work, the truth came out. The patient was found to have insulin pens (needles and syringes) in her room that she was using to cause the hypoglycemic episodes. The *how* was finally explained. But the *why* was dicey.

She admitted to using the pens and even stated that she had done so in the past. However, she tearfully explained her reasoning. She was explicitly told three months ago that she was a pancreas transplant candidate but would never be eligible because of her alcoholism. Although she attempted to quit multiple times, her handle of vodka became increasingly more appealing as her husband's aggressive and verbal behavior worsened.

Quiet, somber and openly questioning the point of life, she simply told us that she wanted to remain in the hospital to avoid her home life. If she stopped drinking (a reasonable assumption while being in the hospital), she would soon get a pancreas transplant. If she went home, she would continue drinking and make herself vulnerable to further domestic abuse.

Although it may be easy to assume this patient is surreptitiously injecting insulin due to her current history of drug use and former profession as a nurse, it is very difficult to think her actions all along were to avoid alcoholism and domestic violence.

This patient taught me a difficult lesson and opened my eyes as to why people may do the things they do. This experience will always remain with me because although her actions are not acceptable, here was a clear opportunity to change this patient's life. Her diagnosis of diabetes ketoacidosis brought her in the hospital, but she was later transferred to the inpatient psychiatry and rehab unit in an effort to cleanse her life. It is premature to say this is the last twist in this patient's life, but it was certainly a story in mine.

Questions

1. What do you think is the "difficult lesson" that the author learned in this story? How do you think it changed the way he approached the care of the patient?

2. The author describes this patient's actions as unacceptable but understandable. Do you think patients are to blame for actions that are detrimental to their health? How would you approach this patient if you were in the author's shoes?

3. How can understanding a patient's seemingly incomprehensible actions lead to more compassionate care?

—Theresa Yang

To the Man with Flowers

October 25, 2013

Sasha Yakhkind
University of South Florida Morsani College of Medicine
Class of 2015

T O THE MAN WITH flowers that I met on my way out of the ICU:
You came up to me and told me how grateful you were to all of the doctors in this place, for how well they treated you and your wife.

You were holding bright red, maybe pink and yellow flowers with gold ribbon in clear wrap. You had grey hair and a kind smile. I said something like, "That's so wonderful, I am glad you had a good experience," and then looked to my left.

My attending physician was far enough down the hall to have already looked back and yelled at me with his eyes to hurry up.

I am sorry that I could not stay and talk. Sharing that moment with you made me feel warm, and I want to thank you for that.

For the rest of the day, I endured a lecture on efficiency.

Despite our common intentions, I observe so many contradictions in medicine. Care, but don't care too much. Follow 11 patients and get enough sleep to make good decisions about their care. Lecture a patient on diabetes, gorge on donuts in the break room, and then roll your eyes at the patient who won't lose weight.

Three months into my third year of medical school, I am not sure what to make of this. I know that I still want to stop in the hallway and say thank you to the man who tells me about his wife's care. I know that I one day hope to perfectly manage 11 patients *and* get enough sleep. I also know that I love sweets and don't know how to effectively talk to patients about their weight.

I guess this is why I am still a student.

Questions

1. In addition to the contradictions the author mentioned, what other hypocrisies or paradoxes in medicine have you witnessed?

2. What steps can medical students take to avoid becoming hypocritical and cynical with their own patients?

3. The author concludes with "I guess this is why I am still a student." Is it reasonable to expect that doctors many years into practice are past such issues themselves? How can caregivers strive to improve their own health while taking care of patients?

—Brent Schnipke

The Little One

November 21, 2013

Eric Ballon-Landa
University of California Irvine School of Medicine
Class of 2015

INTO THE ROOM I hear him come. Above me, his head appears. Then, with blue plastic hands and a dangling toy, he starts poking at me. He lays his hands on my head, then wipes the goop from my face. He shines a light in my eyes and then in my mouth. He prods my neck, then holds the dangling toy against my chest — first here, then there, and listens. He squishes my belly, flips me on my side, runs his fingers down my back, checks my diaper, tickles my feet, pats my head. His eyes smile. I can't see behind his mask, but I think his mouth is smiling, too. He coos something I cannot understand. Then he is gone. The ceiling is back.

—

Into the room I go, calling "Hello!" and "Good morning!", expecting that a mother will emerge from the closed bathroom door that I pass on my way in, or from the pillow-covered armchair in the far corner. There is a baby in the room, dwarfed by her cradle bed and swaddled in blankets. I approach nervously because I want the mother's permission to examine her. But there are no movements in the room other than these 4.5 kilograms of baby and the drips of her IV fluids. I poke my head into the cradle to look at my little patient.

I had been primed to notice her low-set ears, small head and abnormal belly button, the stigmata of her trisomy 13 chromosomal abnormality. This little 11-month-old girl had been hospitalized for "failure to thrive" — yet I could hardly look past her raucous Einsteinian mane of jet-black hair, or her left hand, covered in a grandmother-knit mitten. The mittened hand is in her mouth, and she smacks her lips against it, sucking rhythmically. Too easily, I pull her hand away from her mouth. With plodding, semiconscious effort, the arm resists gravity and inertia to resume its original place. Her limbs are mostly bone — dangling skin that has almost nothing to protect, unanchored vasculature that has almost nothing to nourish. Her belly is distended and soft, splaying to the sides, and she gurgles and burps constantly, unable to control the formula feedings that is sent through her nasogastric tube every three hours. Who can tell if she is hungry?

I left the room, thinking that the child's mother could probably tell when the little girl was hungry. But over the course of six hospital days, I never met the mother. I never learned the answer to my question. I wondered where the girl's mother could possibly be that was more important than being here. How could a being as vulnerable as this little patient can be left alone and still survive the day, and why would a mother, during brief visits at night, sit idle and let a stranger care for her dying child?

Then I remembered that regardless of the very best intentions, unspeakable amounts of love, or uncontrollable grief — there may be other children to feed, family to support, bills to pay, lives to help live.

Questions

1. Have you found yourself in a position where you needed to take another view of a patient's situation? How would you have reacted if this infant was your patient? Would you have the same perspective as the author toward the patient and her mother, or a different perspective?

2. When examining patients, do you consider the encounter from their point of view? How might that perspective change the way that you interact with patients?

3. If you were to meet this patient's mother after six days of never meeting her, how would you approach her? Would you ask her where she had been during her child's hospital stay, or refrain?

—Melanie Watt

Exam Room 3

January 8, 2014

Jimmy Yan
Schulich School of Medicine & Dentistry
Class of 2015

O F ALL THE SOUNDS I expected to hear as I pushed open the thick door of Examination Room 3, the anguished sobs stopped me in my tracks.

Wide-eyed and mouth agape, I stared. Agonizingly long seconds passed.

"Hello, my name is Jimmy..." My mouth instinctively prattled the standard script I had practiced for the last two years. The woman looked up. Behind a mess of straw-colored hair, her red swollen eyes met mine. Dark streaks of mascara painted her face like a Kabuki mask.

I could feel the sweat forming on my face. "I don't know what to do," the woman wailed between sobs.

But let's rewind a bit. It was my first night in the ER. As a clerk, I conducted the initial history interview and physical exam on patients, and then reported back to discuss assessment and management.

A few hours and several cases later, my confidence began to grow. About three-quarters of the way through the night, I asked my attending Dr. T if there was anyone else I could see.

"Why don't you go see the patient in exam room three? Harris. Jaclyn. She's been waiting for a long time now."

That's how I met Jackie.

Now there I stood, dazed, whatever shred of confidence I had built, gone. Funny how little it takes to bring you back to square one.

My brain moved like molasses. In the neural pathway to my vocal cords, a few synapses fired aimlessly, and words drunkenly staggered out of my mouth. I cringed at the phrasing I used.

Jackie did not notice. She brushed a clump of hair out of her eyes and began to talk.

Over the course of the next hour I followed Jackie through her life. Here and there, I asked questions, clumsy attempts to direct her history. Yet these inquiries fell on deaf ears to Jackie. Gradually, I stopped probing and just went with the flow. I began to listen.

Ears and eyes. Hearing the words of her tragic past, recounting episodes of loss, neglect, molestation and abuse. The nuances of her voice, the trembling of her breath between words, and the sobs that bubbled through while she talked. Seeing her hand clutched around the tear-soaked Kleenex, I could count the veins as they popped out. She shifted back and forth, almost as if it was too painful to sit in one place for too long.

A fog enveloped my mind. *How could I help her?*

Defeated, my mental arsenal bare of options, I nodded along. She soon concluded, capping it off with another desperate plea of help. I muttered "we would look into it," purposely shielding myself with the royal *we*.

Emerging from Exam Room 3, the rest of the department hummed away at its usual pace, completely indifferent to what just transpired. I scanned the bay for Dr. T. I spotted him hunched over a desk, analyzing an abdominal CT.

"Hey Dr. T, I was able to get a history from Mrs. Harris. Do you want to hear it?"

"Sure thing, Jim. Just one second."

He leaned back as if reclining on a La-Z-Boy before a Monday night football match. I reviewed the chart, and told him the stressors in Jackie's life, including an incredibly emotionally abusive partner. I emphasized that she had used the term *suicide*, a word that cowed me when I heard her say it, a few times during the interview.

"She was so upset and kept asking for help over and over again. She did not seem to know what she could do for herself at the moment, and I'm not too sure what I could offer to help her, considering the time of night it is." Dr. T listened and nodded as I wrapped up.

"It certainly sounds like she had many emotional traumas, and honestly, we can't really help her with a lot of that. The emergency room is not the place to heal the wounds that have resulted from so many years of abuse. I'm sure she has some form of PTSD. We can keep her safe and settled here tonight and consult psychiatry in the morning so they can assess her."

I asked Dr. T, "Is that all? What about all that crying? I just didn't know what I could do to help."

"There is never an easy answer here, Jimmy. Sometimes you can solve things. Great. Sometimes you can't, but you know who can. And sometimes it's bigger than you. You're going to have to be comfortable with that feeling of being lost, because it's going to be with you for the long run."

Overhead, fluorescent lights flickered. Dr. T wheeled over to a different computer and opened Jackie's file. He unceremoniously checked a "complete" box. The file disappeared. Swallowed somewhere into the ether of the hospital's digital network, it was as if Jackie ceased to exist.

"Come on Jimmy, let's see bed eight. This will be a good case."

I glanced once more at Jackie's chart. It was covered in furious scribblings of my notes. A feeling of doubt still lingered. I did not like it, but I could not shake it.

With one final sigh, I put the chart back into the drawer and followed.

Questions

1. For those of you in your clinical years: Have you ever found yourself in a situation similar to the author's? How did you respond, and what were your thoughts or feelings at the time?

2. For those of you not yet in your clinical years: Have you ever felt power-less in a situation before, and how did you deal with it? If you were in the author's shoes, would you have done anything differently?

3. What do you think of Dr. T's philosophy of accepting the feeling of being lost?

4. If Jackie's chief complaint had been a mysterious medical ailment, what do you think would have been the extent of her work-up in the emergency department? How will you engage with your patients who have a psychiatric complaint?

—Phyllis Ying

Emotions and Energy in the ICU

January 14, 2014

Lisa Moore
Loyola University Chicago Stritch School of Medicine
Class of 2014

DOING A SUB-INTERNSHIP in the ICU is, well, intense. On the first day, I was completely overwhelmed by seeing so many sick patients, most of whom were sedated, ventilated, and on at least one pressor. In just a few weeks, this came to seem perfectly normal.

However, what continued to stir me were the extreme emotions I saw patients and their families experiencing — I couldn't help but feel those emotions myself. The most difficult day was due to the culmination of three very different encounters.

I began the day reviewing my patients' charts with the hope that this would enable me to answer any questions they might have. I first saw a young man who had intentionally overdosed on antipsychotics. I helped admit him when I was on call just two nights before. I stood at the head of the bed during his intubation, cleaned off vomited charcoal, drew an arterial blood gas, and placed a nasogastric tube and Foley. I felt I had actually participated in saving this man's life and was curious to see him again after my day post-call.

He was angry, still intubated but awake, and frustrated at my inability to understand what he was trying to mouth with his endotracheal tube in place. I offered him a pen and paper. He wrote some inappropriate things. I left, saying that was unnecessary and that we would get the tube out as soon as possible. Surprised by the amount of anger I felt, I took a few deep breaths and proceeded to my next patient.

The next patient was also intubated but was able to squeeze my hand, his other hand constantly held by that of his loving wife. After 67 years of marriage, these two were still best friends. It was so touching to see this that I was reminded of a poem by e. e. cummings entitled "i carry your heart with me(i carry it in." I even worked up the courage to read it to her, awkwardly and loudly because she didn't have her hearing aids and because halfway through I noticed his nurse waiting outside the door.

Later that day we would have a family care conference. The patient's wife and children all seemed surprised when we suggested the need to discuss palliative care and terminal extubation for this 92-year-old gentleman with Parkinson's disease, dysphagia and aspiration pneumonia. The room was filled with tears as the children tried to find the right balance between letting their mother make decisions and supporting her by making the most difficult ones themselves.

My third patient painted the classic picture of acute exacerbation of chronic lung disease: a thin "pink puffer" who was still smoking cigarettes up until this most recent episode. She had been intubated for over a week and we already had a very similar conversation with her family. They were certain she would never want a tracheostomy and PEG tube, so we waited. On my post-call day she had been successfully extubated and I was thrilled to finally hear this woman's voice, to see her more alert, and to see her joyful family.

Three very different stories filled with very different emotions, all on the same morning. Part of my struggle was the feeling that I was simply a bystander. Like some object floating in an ocean, the waves of others' emotions crashed over me so that I felt them as if they were my own, but there was nothing I could do about them. I wasn't the doctor making decisions or answering questions. I wasn't the nurse who had been by the patient's bedside all day. I was just there.

In these difficult moments there was one small thing that helped me to feel like I had a bit of control, like maybe I could make some small contribution or, at the very least, comfort myself. As I walked from one room to the next or sat just outside of the circle of family members, I gently held my left thumb in my right hand and after a minute or two methodically switched from one finger to the next, finally holding the palm of my hand in the other. This is one of the simple hand holding techniques of Jin Shin Jyutsu.

Jin Shin Jyutsu originates from ancient Japanese healing practices and was brought to the United States by Mary Burmeister in the 1950s. It entails placing the hands on oneself or another in specific ways for specific ailments based on energy pathways, much like the energy channels that are thought to be responsible for the benefits of acupuncture in traditional Chinese medicine. Each finger corresponds to one of the emotional and organ pathways of the "five element theory." For example, the thumb corresponds to worry, the stomach and the spleen, while the index finger corresponds to fear, the kidney and the bladder, and so forth.

I imagine you are probably rolling your eyes, if I haven't lost you altogether. I get it. I tend to have the same reaction when the "e" word gets thrown around too much. I learned about Jin Shin Jyutsu at an integrative medicine conference and my knowledge is pretty much limited to that, so I'm certainly in no position to defend the practice or to proclaim its wonders.

At the end of the presentation, one conference attendee asked if the benefits of using this with patients — teaching them hand holds or using other techniques that involve touching the patient — was due to the actual particular hand positions, or simply that it was calming, or that patients feel comforted by their doctor's touch. The presenter brilliantly asked him what he thought. His response? "Well, do a randomized controlled trial if you really want to know, but it doesn't seem all that important to me."

I tend to agree and have found it helpful in situations where it's good to feel like I have a bit more control, at least over my own emotions. In the end, I think the point is that we will experience difficult situations and we won't have time to process everything right on the spot. It's important to have something that helps you to feel grounded, to feel like you are still yourself. This little ritual with ancient roots does the trick for me.

Questions

1. Sometimes as a medical student, our job seems limited to just "being there." How can medical students make a difference by just "being there"?

2. What do you see as the role of meditation and mindfulness in patient care? How about their role in medical education?

3. What methods of self-care have you found helpful? What would you recommend to future medical students on maintaining self-care, even on the busiest days?

—Natalie Wilcox

A Sweet Embrace

February 19, 2014

Zachary Abramson
University of Tennessee Health Science Center
Class of 2014

I READ THE LATEST progress note: "67-year-old male with metastatic lung cancer. Mildly agitated. Pain controlled with morphine."

I walk into a single room to see a frail man looking worn beyond his years. I introduce myself and ask if it is a good time to chat. He looks away and tells me that now is not a good time. I can see he has just received his lunch tray. Fair enough. I would not want to be interrupted while eating lunch. I tell him I will check back in a half-hour.

While I wait, I begin writing my note and under the "subjective" heading I write, "mildly agitated."

Thirty minutes later, I return to find him sleeping, slouched over with his hand in his cake, the fork pristinely clean in its setting, his food untouched. With a loud but pleasant voice, I wake him. He is disoriented. He realizes his hand is dirtied but decides to persevere with lunch. He stumbles, unable to perform the complex twirl and scoop needed to gather spaghetti onto his fork. I offer to help but he declines.

I sit down next to him and grab the newspaper, not wanting to make him self-conscious by watching him eat. I casually flip through the paper, occasionally reciting interesting headlines. Out of the corner of my eye, I can see that a few more attempts with the fork are unsuccessful. I tell him I am just going to get the noodles on the fork but he will do the rest. He struggles still. I grab the fork and bring it to his mouth. He hesitates but then concedes.

Again, I walk away, not wanting to make him feel uncomfortable.

I stroll over to a push-pin board with many cards and letters from loved ones. I see a typed letter that begins, "Dear Dad." I read about lost time, missed opportunities, and a childhood memory of a fancy car from a much simpler time.

I ask him about the fancy car and he smiles. I tell him I am from Detroit and my father once had a '64 Ford Mustang, red with white leather interior. He smiles again and with limited breath says, "Yeah, Detroit has great cars."

We chat about cars and sports as I offer a few more servings; he accepts. I tell him we need to get the nurses to change the television off the soap opera channel. He laughs and tells me that his father likes to watch soap operas.

Looking at him and seeing how old and frail he appears, I am surprised to hear that his father is still alive. Without thinking, I ask how old his father is and I immediately feel regret and shame for reminding him of the years of life he will be missing. Quickly, I tell him how great it is to still have one's father for support. He nods and we continue chatting.

A few more forkfuls and his plate is nearly empty. "I'm full," he says. I look up at the clock and I see that I have to be at a meeting soon. I turn to him and say, "Thank you for allowing me to read your letters. You are clearly loved." His eyes widen and he reaches out with his cake-covered hand to grab mine. We sit hand-in-hand in silence.

I can't remember how the embrace ended, or how exactly I said goodbye, but I remember re-writing my note. Changing "mildly agitated" to "pleasantly engaged" could not possibly capture what transpired.

Questions

1. What strategies were used to build rapport with the patient in this story?

2. How do you think this experience changed the author? How do you think this experience changed the patient?

—Daniel Coleman

Do You Remember?

March 5, 2014

Jimmy Yan
Schulich School of Medicine & Dentistry
Class of 2015

T HERE EXIST, IN TRUTH, three simple words that strike dread into the hearts of every physician:

Do. You. Remember.

This phrase was introduced to me in the middle of first year. I was spending time in my medical student lounge when a link popped up on my newsfeed to a TED talk by Dr. Brian Goldman, an emergency physician from Toronto who hosts the radio show "White Coat Black Art" and who has also authored the book "The Night Shift." In the talk, Dr. Goldman reaches out to the audience about changing the medical culture of silence around making mistakes.[1]

When I watched Dr. Goldman's talk, it was clear that he was haunted by several patient encounters that he would never forget.

Fast forward two years. I'm in a family medicine clinic, trying to learn the ropes of ambulatory medicine. A lot of the exposure here is the "bread and butter" cases: sore throats, fevers, rashes, well baby checks, immunizations — all good for honing in on a consistent approach. The work done by clerks involves history and physicals, contributing to an assessment and management plan, as well as conducting basic procedures. To assure patient safety, we're supervised and things are double- and triple-checked by residents, nurses and the attending physicians. I assumed it was a pretty safe system.

Yet one Wednesday morning when I was just arriving to the clinic, Angie, the team nurse pulled me aside. She had a phone in her hand.

"Hey Jim, *do you remember* Greg Foster?" Her voice was hushed, almost solemn. "He came in yesterday with the sore throat."

Yes, Mr. Foster, 45-years-old; he had a two-week long sore throat and a cough that worsened over the course. He stated that the cough did not bring

163

up much sputum, but did produce a sparse, thin and white mucus. No fever, no shortness of breath, no chest pain. No nocturnal symptoms, but he did feel his voice was hoarse. He was not travelling recently and never smoked. On examination he appeared well, not dyspneic, with an occasional dry sounding cough. His heart sounds were present and normal, and his lung fields sounded clear. Pretty much unremarkable up to his pharynx which did look red and irritated but without any swollen glands or petechiae. All vital signs stable. As per the protocol at our clinic I brought in the attending who conducted his own exam. Satisfied, he suggested I perform a rapid strep test but predicted, correctly, that it would be negative.

"It's good for you to practice doing these things." He said, as Mr. Foster was amenable to the idea with a trainee practicing on him.

In the end we thought he had a case of viral pharyngitis and he would soon recover with some more rest and symptomatic management. Mr. Foster seemed reassured and left, and I logged the case, which the resident also reviewed and signed off on. Later my attending reviewed some clinical pearls for sore throats: the group A Streptococcus pharyngitis guidelines, red flags for more serious conditions, and which diagnoses you want to make sure are ruled out (such as peritonsillar abscesses, cancer and epiglottitis). This is pretty typical on how the cases went for me: straightforward.

So why was Angie asking if I remembered Mr. Foster? A low rumble of dread swelled in the back of my head. *What did I miss?*

"Yes, I remember him. He was here yesterday with a sore throat."

"Yeah, it's his wife calling, she's very upset because he was rushed to the emergency room last night, unable to breathe. He had to be intubated at the hospital and he's stabilized now, but it was dicey for a time. The docs at the ER said that it's epiglottitis, and that we should have caught it earlier."

My heart sank. My mind raced. Thoughts exploding out at once. Many of them expletives.

Frantically I tried to go over the whole encounter in my head again, and analyze it again from another angle. Maybe I could recall what was missed.

Was it the hoarse voice? It had to be an early sign, how could I have overlooked that! Stupid stupid STUPID.

My attending came and settled the issue by stating that this "miss" was not something we could have predicted yesterday. Furthermore, I need not think of this as *my* fault, as there was a whole team of people that were also involved in Mr. Foster's care. Yet for the rest of the day, I was shaken.

I think I understand why physicians hate that phrase. It triggers the mind to become obsessively masochistic. It opens Pandora's Box: doubts in one's abilities, anxiety for the subsequent consequences, and fears for the patients. Once opened they can run rampant. The demands of expecting perfection and being immaculate adds to the stress of facing errors. Phrases like "we should have caught it earlier" implicitly throw the blame on other physicians, and perpetuates the ideation that mistakes happen only for "bad" doctors.

At the same time, it's irresponsible to shrug off mistakes nonchalantly by assuming that these incidents are inevitable. By doing so, especially at the trainee level, we not only lose out at a valuable moment to learn but more so, fail to appreciate the outcomes of our actions on the patients. Working as a clinical clerk is not a sterile bubble for us to just learn and "play doctor," but puts us in an environment to start to learn how the consequences of medical decisions can unfold.

It takes experience to find balance within these moments, where we are reminded of our fallibility, to remain assured in our abilities, yet still humbled by the incident to learn. As a student, I have to accept that mistakes and errors will happen and I should not become paralyzed by my fear of making them.

Do you remember?

Before, I wondered when I would first hear this question, and questioned how I'd react to hearing it.

Now, I guess I'm wondering how many more times I'll hear it before I graduate.

Questions

1. Do *you* remember? Do you remember a time when you made a mistake? How did you react to the realization that a mistake had been made?

2. Has a resident or attending ever discussed a mistake they made with you? What lessons did you learn from this conversation? Has a resident or attending ever discussed with you how and when mistakes should be discussed with patients?

3. Do you believe we should discuss mistakes openly within the medical community? Should we discuss those mistakes outside of the medical community?

4. Do you fear failure? Do you fear making mistakes?

—Aleena Paul

Beta Amyloid Blues

March 12, 2014

Kiersten Pollard
University of Colorado School of Medicine
Class of 2014

In the kitchen on the floor
counting the tiles
Again because the number slips
Like all the other numbers slip
Nothing can be proven this way
or solved
And when you call, you never mean to call
the names you say are not the names
You leave the windows open while the neighbors
try not to see
But sometimes it is pieced together
A quilt like waves in a squall
Electricity the thread
A brilliant moment of remembrance
An aching knowledge of what is lost

It is buried again
a bicycle thrown in the Limmat (or was it the Platte?)
visible only from the bridge
A stranger in your house and picture frames
A mouse in our water maze
O, captive experiment "it's for your own good!"
Forgetting is the cruelest
and yours has made us cruel
But we feed you pancakes and talk about clouds
Sometimes we cry and you see us
as children in sweaters as you struggle to pay the electric bill

It's been a hundred years at least if it's been
no time at all?
Keeping you here with the lights on during the day
We must always wear our glasses
You draw clocks and we set clocks as purposeful compasses
whose needles spin in your vertiginous seas
A meaningless countdown
We contain you here as you leave
for the sake of memories

Questions

1. If the name didn't give away the diagnosis, would you know what this poem was about and why?

2. Is there another meaning to this poem besides the life of a patient with Alzheimer disease? Have you interacted with a person diagnosed with memory dysfunction? If so, reflect on this interaction. How could your next interaction be better?

3. Can you imagine what losing your sense of self, your sense of time, your identity would feel like? What would it feel like to witness a loved one go through this — to forget you, and maybe dislike you for trying to care for them?

—Sam Marguiles

A Story of Love from Psychiatry

March 20, 2014

Manasa Mouli
Tufts University School of Medicine
Class of 2015

THE PATIENT WAS A man in his sixties, sitting in the armchair. His wife was next to him. He was there for his routine appointment with a psychiatrist about his depression, stress and anxiety. A year ago, he had a stroke, followed by a motor vehicle accident. His wife is now his caretaker.

"It's hard to take care of him at home, when I'm at work all day, too," she said. "And he hasn't been sleeping well. He gets up in the middle of the night and then wanders through the house because he's anxious about where he is and he thinks he's trapped in the house. I try to follow him so that he doesn't fall down the stairs or get into the kitchen knife drawer. He doesn't come back to bed. He tries to fight me off."

She looked worn down, like she was under a lot of stress.

Her husband now has mild cognitive impairment and he is frequently unaware of where he is. He doesn't remember much about his past; half of the time, he also doesn't understand much about his current circumstances, except that something is wrong with him and that his body doesn't work the way it used to. His speech is slurred. That combined with his impaired memory and awareness means that most of what he says is either inaccurate or confused.

In spite of seeing many patients like him (or ones that are even worse off) on my psychiatric rotation so far, situations like this are still uncomfortable. I try to remain entirely emotionally detached from patients when I hear their unfortunate stories. Certain things always stand out, though. It is easy to see that he is frustrated that his life is like this now. And when we hear these stories, we sympathize and want to help. It's even easier to see that it hurts his wife more than it affects him.

Sometimes when I'm sitting there listening to patients like this, I have a sudden eerie realization that they were young and happy and in love once.

168

They have an entire life that they have lived, before the accident or stroke or whatever it is that makes them come to your office today. I felt sorry for him, especially because there isn't much we could do to significantly help him cope with his stressors. We can't change his situation.

And I felt so sorry for his wife. It was very obvious that she loves her husband, and to her, taking care of him was a part of her commitment to the marriage. I don't personally know what that kind of commitment is like, but it seemed difficult to take that on and continue shouldering the responsibilities when her husband is not going to be contributing to the relationship in the same way anymore, and when it might not feel like an equal partnership to her anymore. They probably did not anticipate this turn in their lives on the day they got married.

Then he started to speak in mumbling sentences about his years spent working and with his family.

"I ... was a ... engineer. I loved it... And..." he trailed off. But he patted his wife on the arm once, and I'd like to think that he was showing his appreciation for his wife, even if he couldn't express it in any other way.

The patient could not answer any of the doctor's questions. He couldn't understand the question, couldn't verbalize the answer, or just didn't remember things anymore. His wife answered on his behalf. Towards the end of the visit, the doctor tested the patient's memory, cognition, language skills and awareness. He asked him to spell "w-o-r-l-d" backwards, count from one to 10, and then he asked him to write a sentence on a piece of paper. Any sentence that the patient could form and that he wanted to write. He shakily scribbled something down. Before he handed it to the doctor, I saw what it said.

"I love my wife."

The wife didn't see what he had written down before he handed it over to his doctor. But I hope she figured it out anyways.

Questions

1. The author reflects on the history of a patient before he comes to the office. Do you ever find yourself thinking about what a patient may have been like before his or her illness? Does that perspective influence your approach to the patient?

2. In patients who have lost their ability to communicate through "standard" means — talking, writing, sign language — how can you assess their feelings and what they do and do not understand? Do you find yourself paying attention to nonverbal cues or body language to interpret a patient encounter? Is this an effective way to deal with this communication barrier? Why or why not?

3. Patients' families are often forced into the role of "caretaker" due to a loved one's unexpected illness. Do you think it is the physician's responsibility to care for the caretaker in addition to the patient? If so, how can that be achieved?

—Claire Drom

Eyes: A Reflection from the First Month of Clerkships

August 6, 2014

Sanjay Salgado
Weill Cornell Medical College
Class of 2015

IN 1984, IN THE MIDST of fleeing the Soviet invasion of Afghanistan, a young girl agreed to pose for a photo. In her short life, she had survived the carpet bombings that claimed the lives of her parents, trekked through mountains to escape her war-torn home, and struggled to adjust to life amongst a sea of other refugees — but she had never been photographed. Restricted by her religion from smiling at a male photographer, she gazed into the camera for an instant before returning to a life of survival — the photographer never even got her name. That instant, however, quickly became the most famous *National Geographic* photo in the history of the magazine, known simply as "The Afghan Girl." As *National Geographic* put it, "Her eyes are sea green. They are haunted and haunting, and in them, you can read the tragedy."

In the first two years of medical school, we are taught the physiology and pathophysiology of the eyes. We learn how to use light to measure the reactivity of pupils, and study how and where those signals are processed in brain. We memorize all the extraocular muscles, where they originate and attach, and how to interpret deficiencies in gaze. We learn a rainbow of pathology, creating knee-jerk differentials for red, yellow and blue sclera. And like everything else we study in the first two years, we then take an exam and move on to the next organ system, with most of us (except perhaps the future ophthalmologists) surmising that we've learned everything we need to know about the eyes.

It's not until we finally reach the wards that it becomes clear that there is an entire hidden curriculum devoted to deciphering a patient's eyes. My patients taught me the basics.

A stoic Chinese immigrant, fluent only in her native language of Mandarin, was in a daily struggle to contain the insurmountable pain caused by

171

her cholangiocarcinoma. She managed her disease with an expressionless resolve, burying her emotions far from the surface. As she became ascitic and the pain grew, her eyes began betraying her guise, giving me a real glimpse into her suffering. Eventually, she relented and agreed to a therapeutic paracentesis. With each liter of fluid removed, relief washed over her. That afternoon, four liters lighter, she spoke English to me for the first and only time, her eyes wide with sincerity: *thank you.*

An elderly woman was admitted for shortness of breath and subsequently diagnosed with advanced metastatic lung cancer, remaining on the floor for the entire month my team was on service. She progressively found it harder to move, harder to breathe, harder to speak. She considered herself a fighter, insisting on anything we could do to make her live longer, and always reminding us that she wasn't ready to say goodbye just yet. On the general medicine floor, where so many patients are discharged within days, a month is akin to an eternity — we were with her for so long, she started referring to us as her "hospital family." At the end of the month, the teams turned over. As we explained to her that a new family would be coming to take care of her, her eyes filled with a new pain: abandonment. "I thought you would be with me until the end," were the only words she could muster. The day the new team began its rotation, she passed away.

In the cardiac intensive care unit, I cared for a ex-correctional officer who was admitted for heart failure. A gregarious Brooklynite, she always managed to be cheerful — and in a place like the CCU, cheer is usually in short supply. The team always saw her first or last — first if we needed a joke to start the day, or last if we needed to lift our spirits after rounds. Two days before she was to be discharged, my fellow medical student and I sat with her during dinner, as a means of saying goodbye. We never thought we would be the last people to share a meal with her. We arrived the next morning to a situation that had spiraled beyond hope — our patient developed an inexplicable lactic acidosis, and was suddenly not expected to make it through the day.

Ten minutes into morning rounds, the bells started.

Whenever we walk into a room, eye contact is the first thing we notice. But for physicians, especially in a place like an ICU, there is an overwhelming sense of dread when we walk into a room and a patient doesn't meet our gaze. Our voices become raised to the point of shouting, our hands find themselves shaking the patient for any response, and amongst a tidal wave of adrenaline, time slows to a crawl.

For all of medicine's technological advances, the basic idea behind a code is brutally simple. When a patient's heart stops working, our hands do its work. As we started compressions, desperately trying to get blood to the brain, her eyes opened. They darted throughout room, eventually settling on me. Twelve hours ago, she had given me a wink and asked jokingly the odds the doctors would agree to let her go skydiving. Now her eyes were full of horror.

Studies have shown that when people die, they want to go peacefully, passing from this life surrounded by their family and loved ones. No one wants to imagine dying naked in a room full of doctors forcing air into their lungs and coercing their hearts to beat. And while for that first round, we stabilized her, her acidosis was a opponent we knew we had no chance of beating. Her family, after watching what we did to keep her alive, asked us to not to intervene the next time. A half hour later, she died, in the way most of us wish to go.

Seventeen years after the picture of "The Afghan Girl" was taken, the photographer returned to Pakistan, searching for the that nameless girl with the piercing green eyes. They eventually found her living in the mountains near Tora Bora. She had never seen the picture of herself, nor could she understand how her eyes captivated the world. Living though a decades old conflict that took over two million lives, she was asked how she managed to survive. "It was," she said, "the will of God."

As doctors, we become used to the seeing death creep up on our patients. It is never easy to watch our patients slowly succumb, but time lets us admit there is nothing more we can do, and allows us to ensure they pass away in comfort. When a patient dies suddenly, we carry a heavier load of doubt. *Why didn't we know? Could we have saved her?* Trying to relieve some of this burden, I went to the autopsy of my ICU patient. As we laid her body on the table, her eyes were open. That was the first time I looked into a patient's eyes after death.

I had to close them.

Questions

1. Discuss the nonverbal ways in which patients communicate their needs and concerns with their care providers.

2. Reflect on a time when you felt burdened by the care that was provided to a patient. Did you or your team do too little? Too much?

3. We have often heard the phrase, "the eyes are the windows to the soul." Of all the parts that make up the human body, why do you think we place such emphasis on the eyes?

—Aleena Paul

We Lost It: A Story of Surgical Error

November 19, 2014

Dacia Russell
Ohio State University College of Medicine
Class of 2015

I WILL ADMIT TO being an "OR avoider" — albeit, one who is certainly in awe of the stylized pageantry of sterile armor adornment. In the operating room, safe spaces are demarcated by mere inches. Rest your hand beyond the thresholds monitored by the scrub techs and you are deemed a threat to a clean procedure. Gesturing in ways that are otherwise socially advantageous gives new territory to harmful bacteria that threaten favorable outcomes.

As third-year medical students, we are taught patient safety in the instruction we receive on behaviors that adhere to evidence-based guidelines for minimizing surgical complications. This education undeniably evolves with our understanding of the science and systems that underline medical practice. For me, a specific OR experience remarkably transformed and accelerated my education in patient safety. Witnessing and participating in the unfolding of a medical error made me rethink the resources necessary and available for safe medical decision-making.

Our case was a laparoscopic inguinal hernia repair. Nothing in the team's preoperative routine diverged from the customs designed to optimize surgical results. We reviewed the patient's chart to confirm that the proper procedure with the right location would be performed for the correct person. Surgical sites were marked. Consent was reiterated and lingering questions were answered. Once in the OR, a time-out ensued. Sterile drapes were positioned. We began, seemingly without event.

Shallow anatomical planes defined the workspace. To reach from abdomen to groin, small incisions were made, into which even smaller trocars were placed. Technical success required delicate coordination between surgeon, equipment and fascia. The torn tissue arose in view prompting the scrub tech to offer a needle for the repair. A few millimeters of steeply curved medical technology, the needle seemed an odd match for the exacting straightness of the trocar. The surgeon reflexively shared this sentiment. "This needle won't fit." But with a curious reversal of opinion bolstered by an unobserved expression of logic, the needle was advanced. And it complied with stiff walls of the trocar. But did it emerge unchanged? Dissatisfied with the progress after several turns of the needle, the surgeon pulled back on the anchoring suture. Only its frayed end returned. The needle was lost in the patient.

The pivot from progress to error in our case was the consequence of multiple factors. We were time pressured. Several complex cases were scheduled after our case, and regiment loomed large in the stated objectives of the team. We were performance pressured. The surgeon had only completed a few inguinal hernia repairs laparoscopically. Moreover, the relative newness of the procedure certainly extended to me as well as the assisting senior resident who was a relative novice with these procedures. We were decision pressured. We had delayed seeking assistance at key junctures. Thus, procedural unfamiliarity and uncertainty stood in the stead of seasoned guidance that might have reformed aberrant decisions.

These challenges are certainly not novel. But our preparation and impulses could most favorably be described as inadequate. Reflecting on our situation and reviewing patient safety literature, several mechanisms stand out as potential safety measures. For one, tethering individual accountability to a bias for inquiry transforms any moment of participation into a platform for turnaround. Practically, this means that we promptly ask questions and seek expertise as we become more uncertain. Culturally, this demands that we work to dismantle norms that concentrate authority in any one person or in any one paradigm. Secondly, investing in ritualized protocols and appropriate interruptions that include equipment checklists and intraoperative time-outs are powerful add-ons to reduce risk. These practices help eliminate unneeded patient risks and work to protect the patient. Lastly, empowering health care teams with viable resources to manage workflow represents a formidable stake in protecting patients. Such resources can be articulated from multiple perspectives. That is, institutions can establish workload management policies, practitioners can advocate for optimal staffing, and even national authorities can weigh in with analysis of protocols that address safety in workflow.

Ultimately, a senior surgeon was called for guidance. Multiple rounds of imaging were completed. The consensus of data gathered and expertise elicited settled on making an open abdominal incision. Subsequently, the needle was recovered. The attending surgeon and senior partner openly discussed their intention to fully disclose the error to the patient and patient's family. Unfortunately, I was not able to see the patient in recovery and gauge his reaction to the phalanx of staples meandering on his abdomen. Nor was I privy to the disclosure between surgeon and patient where the events of the surgery were recounted. My hope is that all was ultimately well.

The lessons from this case have motivated me to strike new commitments to patient safety. I was encouraged by the culture of safety and disclosure that flanked our case. This culture has been nurtured through years of patient safety scholarship and grooming leaders who are open and willing to learn from their organization's mistakes. Yet, there were deficiencies in our approach that reveal avenues for sustained improvement. As I contemplate integrating technology with the norms of medical practice, I am thus driven to advocate for a framework where questions are viewed as assets, pooled expertise is the default for tackling uncertainty and professional accountability includes the authority to command resources to optimize safety.

Questions

1. Should a patient be made aware of situations like those described in this passage, even if the outcome is positive?

2. New technologies are often introduced into medicine with the intention of improving patient safety. However, these same technologies can be sources of error as they are integrated into practice. What steps can be taken to ensure safe adoption of these innovations?

3. Is more technology always better? Think of a time you observed patient care being compromised because of the use of "advanced technology."

—Kate Joyce

How to Make Challah: The Jewish Octopus

December 19, 2014

Ajay Koti
University of South Florida Morsani College of Medicine
Class of 2017

C HALLAH BREAD IS traditionally prepared for Jewish holidays and the Sabbath. We made ours on a Wednesday night.

Helen and Marie stare warily from their wheelchairs as a dozen medical students file into the retirement home lounge, toting tubs of flour and challah dough. "We're not playing bingo?" Helen asks, looking disappointed, as students and octogenarians begin matching up for the evening. (She won fifty cents last time.)

"Where are you all from?" Marie asks. I tell her we are students from the medical school, which seems to please her.

"I really admire people doing that. My mother was a nurse, you know."

"What specialty?" I ask.

"Family medicine," she replies, smiling approvingly.

The dough is passed out and we roll it into ropes, mashing them together at one end. In its unwoven state, the challah looks like a kind of octopus. A Jewish octopus — "Oy," Marie says, shaking her head at the thought.

Helen, meanwhile, is having difficulty. Her hands tremble as she attempts to braid the ropes. "I didn't know we were doing this. I thought we were playing bingo." My own efforts to assist are decidedly unhelpful, and we assemble what must be the world's most pitiful challah. "Not exactly the dynamic duo, are we?" Marie looked on bemusedly. She had been a baker at a school cafeteria in the past; the students never tired of her chocolate chip cookies.

We keep braiding, passing strands of dough over and around each other. Marie scans the students around the room and taps my shoulder, her brow furrowed. "Where are you all from?" I am familiar to her, but she can't quite place me.

After a coating of egg wash and sesame seeds, the woven challahs are whisked to the oven, and the room is transformed. Seniors who would otherwise be in the throes of bingo night are sharing stories with new friends. Marie misses the snowy winters of her Midwestern hometown, where she remembers making snow angels. Helen has a daughter, Lily, who works in advertising. Lily takes her mother to lunch every week. "I'm going to give her my challah," she resolves.

Marie can't remember the last time her daughter visited.

Helen points out one of the facility's administrators, a virile man with thick forearms, who the residents have dubbed 'Stan the Man.'

"Why do you call him that?" I tease. Helen shoots back, "Just look at him!"

Marie drifts away, her eyes glazed over. Turning back to me, she asks, "Where are you from?"

I try another tack — "Pennsylvania." She smiles and gestures to the room. "No, no. I mean, where are you all from?" I am reminded that diseases like Alzheimer's and dementia affect family and friends just as much as they affect patients. But this principle is now visceral to me as I repeat that we are from USF, that we are medical students, and that I am specializing in family medicine.

"That's good, you know? I really admire people who do that. You know, my mother was a nurse."

The oven door opens and the air is thick with the aroma of fresh bread. Helen and Marie's lopsided creations are more elegant in their finished form.

Helen chews on a piece of challah and closes her eyes in satisfaction. She asks if I'd like to take her challah home, until I ask her about Lily. "That's right, I forgot. I'll give it to Lily." Marie looks at me, with more urgency this time. "Where are you all from?"

The evening ends with a group picture, and a woman who was likely student body president in her time directs her fellow residents into formation, somewhat overzealously. "No, no, you stand over *here*," she shrills at a sleepy-looking man in suspenders. Helen and Marie look on quizzically. "Who put her in charge?" Helen whispers, proof that high school never really ends.

The facility staff arrives to escort residents to their rooms, and I say my goodbye to Marie and Helen. An aide wheels Helen toward the hallway. "Did you bake that for me?"

Helen stares at the still-warm bread in her lap. There is something she is supposed to do with it. Then she offers it to the aide, who tears off a bite. "Delicious!"

Helen grins, and they head off down the hallway.

On the drive home, we remembered stories of the people we met that night. One gentleman proudly touted his Ohio roots, yet his front door displayed a placard that read: 'Don't Mess with Texas.' (Whether this is a reflection on Texas or Ohio is another debate entirely.) I remembered Marie's confusion, the empty look in her eyes. Helen's unsteady hands. In those gnarled, trembling hands I could see those of my grandmother, shaking as she buttons her cardigan, as she guides a steaming cup of tea to her lips. I can hear the bangles on her wrist jingling as she sips. For years, she has asked me, "When you are a physician, can you fix my hands?"

At the very least, we can bake some bread.

Questions

1. Think of an instance when a patient reminded you of a family member. Did you treat this patient differently? Why?

2. What is the difference between the care we give to patients and the care we give to family?

3. Name ways in which you can bridge the gap between "patient care" and "care for patients."

—Sasha Yakhkind

Why I Am in the Room

January 23, 2015

Katie Taylor
Icahn School of Medicine at Mount Sinai
Class of 2016

S HE ASKED ME if I was from New York. I told her I wasn't. I was from California, actually, but enjoying myself in New York City while I was here. I asked her where she grew up. She said Brooklyn. She asked to see my referral card. I asked her to clarify. She said she wanted to see my referral card. For coming here. And did the super know I was here? Where *was* my card?

I was on a home visit as part of my internal medicine clerkship. We were visiting five home-bound patients today, and Mrs. B, who was the second of our visits, was less than delighted that we had made our way to her living room.

"You know, it is rude to show up unannounced," she explains. I told her that her husband and health aide had known we were coming. I thought about adding that she had also probably known, for a brief time.

Mrs. B is wearing a tropical muumuu. Her short gray hair had been wetted and combed backwards. She has three remaining teeth, which all neighbor one another. Her lips cave around her gums, mostly, except where the last few hang on.

We inspect Mrs. B's swollen ankles and then examine a dry patch of skin on her right elbow. I take her blood pressure, which is normal, and her pulse, which bounds along as even as ever. The attending steps out to call Mrs. B's husband.

Mrs. B starts to pick at her elbow. Her aide tells her to let it be and moves toward her. Mrs. B grabs the aide's forearm with her bulbous, arthritic hands and, with a growl, tries to bite, her three teeth looking like a cartoon baby's against the black of her open, agape mouth. The aide patiently pulls her arm lower, Mrs. B's atrophied muscles unable to compete in this match of strength. Mrs. B growls and tries to bite again.

"That is not very nice, Mrs. B," her aide says, pulling her arm entirely away. I ask if Mrs. B had ever actually bit her, to which Mrs. B interjects that SHE DOES NOT BITE!

I do not want to linger here. I am scared of this woman. I imagine her lunging at me, leading with a few-toothed snarl. I find her a terrifying exemplar of what age does to a mind. I imagine what Mr. B looks like, what his temperament must be like. What it is like coming home to your lifelong partner, now warped by dementia, a washed and combed version of whoever she once was.

"Where is your card?" Mrs. B asks me. "I am going to the police. I will call them!" I explain that her doctor visits every two months. I am a student visiting just this time. "I will call the police," she threatens again. Had I not heard her? I repeat what I have just told her. She repeats what she has just threatened.

"Help! HELP! HELP! HEEEEEELLLLLPPPPPP! Someone help me!" Her fear has spilled over into action. She wails over my continued explanations, so I sit in silence as she pleas with anyone passing by to help. To the neighbors, I suppose. Or to the god she believes in, perhaps. When she finally stops, she looks about to cry.

I am ill-prepared for her punishing, unremitting perception of reality. I cannot calm her, or right her mind. Unable to convince the other, we sit in silence, until a giant, towering grandfather clock standing across the room goes off. It is twelve o'clock, so we are lucky enough to witness its full, timely concerto.

"What an amazing sound," I say.

"You are such a phony. Do you know that?" this elderly Holden Caulfield asks. After all, how can one *bear* the small talk of a burglar? She dives back into another round of threats and screams.

Finally, the attending returns, and we ready to leave, for which I am relieved. I wonder how Mr. B deals with the daily howls.

Or, perhaps this only happens once every two months, when strangers barge inward and demand to squeeze her arms, pinch her ankles and prod her belly. For however scared I was, I was able to appreciate the relationship and roles of each person in the tableau of her living room. She is the one left to fend off the intruders, to first politely inform them of their indiscretions, and then, when that doesn't work, scream for help. Is everyone else mad? There are intruders and phonies in every direction!

We head down the hall. Her muffled wails drift towards us as the elevator climbs upwards. My fear and unease and distress at our meeting thaw into a sadness, for a life and personality distorted by dementia. And that sadness soon ebbs into a compassion for a last stage of life filled with constant and profound fearfulness. Mrs. B had gifted me a deep appreciation of something I had never considered — a gratitude for knowing why I am in the room.

Questions

1. What network of people are affected when someone has dementia?

2. What social supports can clinicians provide for families of patients with dementia? Have you ever seen any of these employed? Did they work for the patient and their family? Why or why not?

3. The home visit is an archaic and ineffective process. Agree or disagree, and explain your reasoning.

4. Have you ever experienced feelings of dislike, fear or repulsion when taking care of patients? How did you react to those feelings? Would you react in the same way as the author did toward her patient?

—Natalie Wilcox

Fading Memories of Love and Martinis

January 27, 2015

Joshua Niforatos
Cleveland Clinic Lerner College of Medicine
Class of 2019

"IF I BEGIN TO repeat myself, just tell me. I have Alzheimer's. At least, I think I do," the elderly gentleman said with a smile.

This elderly patient of mine was a jovial gentleman and in fantastic shape with unremarkable vitals on physical examination. If it was not for his diagnosis of Alzheimer's disease, the physical and emotional state of this patient given his age is nothing less than enviable.

A narrative filled with stories emblematic of living throughout the mid-1900s, he described to me the fading memory of lovers and loved ones while looking at pictures of them in his wallet. The sight of their faces can, at least for now, trigger memories of the past for him: memories of joy and sorrow, of love and lost, of mountaintop and valley experiences.

I noticed in the periphery of my vision a painting by Vincent Van Gogh that I had once seen while on a Valentine's Day date at the Boston Museum of Fine Art. As I glanced at the painting on the exam room wall, I recognized it as Van Gogh's 1890 "House at Auvres." After leaving the asylum at Saint-Rémy in France in 1890, Van Gogh made his way to Auvers-sur-Oise, which is north of Paris. Despite Van Gogh's depression while at Auvres, he managed to produce around 100 pieces of art in 70 days.

As I recalled these memories of a date and the brilliance of the last two months of van Gogh's life in the context of my patient's inability to remember so many precious details of his past, I became overwhelmed with the fear of fading memories and experienced what psychiatrist-anthropologist Arthur Kleinman refers to as the "powerful, enervating anxiety created by the limits of our control over our small worlds and even over our inner-selves."[1]

"Are you a gin or vodka guy?" he said in excitement as he seemed to recall an all-but-faded memory from his past.

"Gin. Why?" I asked.

"On that piece of paper, take down the following recipe for my famous martini," he said on the edge of his seat.

My patient began to describe the intricacies related to the art of mixing drinks in astounding detail. After a few minutes, however, he became forgetful of what he was talking about and I used this opportunity to continue the medical history.

I realized during the disconnected memories of this patient that the powerful, enervating anxiety I was feeling was due to the discomfort that comes with the idea of being faced with one's mortality. We often think of mortality in terms of physical death but mortality can also be relational and historical death — an inability to recall one's past, respond to one's present and to project hope onto one's future.

The ominous words of Rosencrantz from British playwright Tom Stoppard's "Rosencrantz and Guildenstern Are Dead" concerning the moment one becomes aware of mortality distracted me: "We must be born with an intuition of mortality. Before we know the words for it, before we know that there are words, out we come, bloodied and squalling with the knowledge that for all the compasses in the world, there's only one direction, and time is its only measure."[2]

My patient was aware of the direction and measure of his compass, which was the reason why he was wrapping up loose ends in his life while he still could. Van Gogh seemed to be aware of his inability to reconcile his larvate epilepsy with a night sky that was no longer starry. Both my patient and Van Gogh were in touch with difficulties I currently chose to ignore because of the existential difficulty they would pose. As medical students we are taught to demonstrate empathy during the medical history, yet we are not always given the tools on how to handle enervating anxiety that comes with being vicariously introspective.

"Alright, sir, I'll go talk with Dr. Green about our conversation and we'll come back and try to address your concerns today."

"Do you ever take a break?" he laughed while leaning forward to give me a pat on the knee.

"Occasionally," I smiled back.

"Oh, then let me tell you how to make a good martini!" The excitement was beaming from his face as he seemed to temporarily re-remember one of the joys of these fading memories of love and martinis, not recalling that he had given me the recipe a few minutes earlier.

"I'd love to hear it, sir."

Questions

1. The author mentions different 'forms' of mortality such as physical death, emotional death and relational death. Addressing these potentialities is unnerving. Have you ever confronted your own mortality? If so, when and how? How can the confrontation of your own mortality help you address those same feelings in your patients?

2. Imagine you are faced with imminent death, but you are allowed one final conversation. With whom would you choose to have it? What is the one memory that you have that you would wish to pass on to that person? Why?

—Brent Bjornsen

M/R/G
March 2, 2015

Steven Lange
Albany Medical College
Class of 2017

Stunted by the shadow of its flow
pouring, rumbling in a lifelong swing
through the raging heart of darkness rings
the steadfast drip: a weak and lonely bruit,
and pitting insult in the turbid skin
with shocking faults to grimly thinning walls
the fallen house still stands; the flagging strands
and edematous sands chafe the burning soles.
Statuesque, he shifts his swollen ruin
laying, turning to dispel the pain
the tightened breath, the hypercapnic brain;
and ushering the mad errata
speaks to the miscellaneous shapes:
a reaction to digoxin
or the amorphous figures fidgeting
with drugs and dials, while he ponders
the pages never written, the stubborn weight
of things abandoned and retained,
the drinks that oft were drunk
and clouds that moped behind the pelting rain
and out of hiding came to bear his fears —
plaques amassing in the tired works
from lipid laden in the careless years.
The children stake their futures,
the old remit their past
to live with wicked fibrillations
while the former pave their path

without the wet, tachypneic throes
breathing without the toll of having
chests like barrels or lungs iron-clad.
Mere words remembered, mentioned in the haste
of fateful falls and bobbing heads —
regurgitations in lopsided beds —
and grudging workers heeding muffled calls
awake physicians to a mourning place:
the red pools surging on this mount
and blue, congested hearts — still — waiting — count
S1, S2, the ominous swishing tune,
pouring out their hollow sounds, commonly found
to be more brisk than the *cor* permits
while time moves slowly through relentless fits.
They lumber towards the crowded doors
where revolutions start and finish;
the vacant, *whooshing* valves emitting
lives half-lived, binged, or lived too much;
aged perversely by their eating,
growing clammy to the touch,
and worsened by persistent sitting,
indicted by the minor scut
that filled those pipes in silent smite
and tasked the chambers, flogged the host
with the extremities of stresses,
as they reimbursed organic messes.
The telltale heart uprooted from its floor
to feel its final filling phase no more.
And running on motors and emotions,
bombshells and reverberations,
holosytolic and post-Romantic,
a heart devoid of delectations
strives in denial of a means
to turn back time, to have its body cleaned
of stagnancy and ripe transgressions,
engaging at last the right to life
to a last resort or forceful fight
replayed in echoes, stents, and rays,
ACEs and ARBs and conduction delays.
And always a minute behind
gasping at the gate, this ponderous form of late
finds solace in the daily grind: a way
of catching one's breath, "yourself" (you jest);
but misplaced beats mistake their step
and fail to grant a moment yet

that does not cause a gasp.
Quoted by your pleural bases
and mindful of the AV gap,
your family surrounds the bed
with worried thoughts now racing through their heads,
with despondent but more youthful faces,
watching this inconsequential test
demonstrate the war beneath your chest,
where crests and troughs affirm the case
and imminent need of permanent rest
during your final excursion
into ventricular rhythm.

Questions

1. In the pair of pieces by this author, M/R/G and EKG Calamity (page 7), the author describes well-functioning and failing hearts. Discuss how the author highlighted aspects of patients' lives by focusing on their hearts. What imagery does the author use to showcase health and to portray disease?

2. In one piece, the author focuses on the anatomy of the heart; in the other, the author places the heart in the context of the suffering patient. How do you think your perception of anatomy will change or has changed from gross anatomy dissection to real patients? Is this perceptual change important?

3. In both poems, the author interlaces rich emotional language into the heart's repetitive physiology. What emotions did you feel during gross anatomy dissection? How were those emotions similar to or different from the emotions you feel when treating patients?

—Aleena Paul

The Lady in Red

March 13, 2015

Lisa Podolsky
FIU Herbert Wertheim College of Medicine
Class of 2016

HER STORY STARTED pretty similarly to any other patient I had over the past week and a half since starting my family medicine rotation. The nurse told me she had another patient who was checking in. I asked her for the name and began looking up the previous clinical notes and labs in the computer while waiting for her arrival from registration. She had a history of arthritis, GERD and uncontrolled diabetes — all diagnoses I had become comfortable discussing with patients. Her last follow-up note indicated a plan to obtain x-rays for her knee pain, metformin for her diabetes, and health maintenance screenings in the upcoming year. Although I was confused that she did not have a visit in the previous nine months, I simply assumed she would have an x-ray with some answers and hopefully have lowered her glucose at least below her previous measurement of over 400.

I was wrong.

The nurse walked in with a lady in gold shoes and a head-to-toe red outfit. As I was waiting for the nurse to finish taking her vitals, this lady in red began expressing her frustration at how long it took to get an appointment, and her worries that her J02 card expired that day. (A J02 card is a classification given out to Miami-Dade residents living under the federal poverty level, providing them with hospital services without charge.) With her bag of Easter candies and soda in hand, she was asking us to check her glucose levels, since she was concerned how high they were at the last visit. I was wondering why she was eating chocolate and drinking soda if she was concerned about her sugar level; I thought this would clearly be a visit filled with patient education about diabetes, glycemic index and healthier eating habits. As soon as the patient's vitals were finished, the lady in red started listing off her problems to me — vaginal itching, acid reflux, "sugars," loss of feeling in her hand, breast pain, and the list went on.

When I started asking about each complaint individually, I could not understand how someone had gone unseen with so many symptoms, each of them unaddressed and worsening over the past year. How could a patient have vaginal itching and discharge for over a year? How could a patient feel pain and a lump in her breast without telling someone? How could someone with a previous glucose over 400 stop her metformin? I remember asking her to remove her shoes to check for ulcers, and immediately the smell of the fungal infections in her toenails filled the room. However, with each complaint more of the story began to come together. She was homeless and could no longer afford Nexium; water and baking soda would have to do for her reflux. If her sister needed to have her toes amputated because her diabetes was so bad, why wasn't the patient more concerned about her own diet? The candy only cost 50 cents and her food stamps had run out. But why did she stop the metformin if it's free from Publix? She lost her bus card and had no way to get to Publix.

With each part of the story, her depression showed through more and more. She tried to commit suicide two months ago, but it didn't work; she felt she even failed at dying. She didn't understand why god kept letting her wake up each morning. Although I'd seen patients with depression most days since I started my rotation, I had never discussed previous suicide attempts. She was the second patient ever to cry to me, and the first with a previous suicide attempt. I had never seen such hopelessness, and it broke my heart.

Our approach had to change. We were no longer concerned about addressing her acid reflux, arthritis or health maintenance. Our priorities had to be about addressing the most imminent and extreme issues — her suicide attempt and controlling her diabetes. We had to mobilize the nurses and pharmacy in order to obtain her free metformin there in the clinic that day, before the pharmacy closed in a half hour and her JO2 coverage ran out, and before she fell to the risk of requiring amputation like her sister. Next step, refer her to a psychiatrist — but that costs money. We discussed with her exactly how she could obtain a homeless Jackson Card, so all referrals, tests and medications would be free and we could see her again.

By the end of the visit I felt I had just come out of a rushed whirlwind tunnel. Although our assessment and plan at the end of the visit didn't address everything we would have wanted to at the beginning of the visit, I know we helped this patient. From her I learned to prioritize a patient's problems, looking at the resources they have, and working with what you can. Referring for x-rays or discussing diet wouldn't have mattered — she couldn't afford x-rays and she ate what she could get. By the end of this one visit, I learned unforgettable lessons. I learned how to better support an overwhelmed patient who felt hopeless, as well as how to ask for help from the nurses, pharmacist, and finance department to address extreme situations. No matter the situation in life, you always have to be adaptable to change and listen for the subtle comments. By listening to the little comments about her walking to the clinic, and about her missing her family, we were able to probe further into her depression.

Medicine is an ever-changing field, whether it's the patients, guidelines, medications or scientific discoveries. Medicine requires knowing how to adapt to change by knowing the whole story, and then working with the resources available. On the seventh day of my family medicine clerkship, the lady in red helped teach me those skills.

Questions

1. Discuss the ways in which the author was able to provide compassionate care for her patient.

2. Sometimes patients arrive with more issues and concerns than the physician can possibly address in one visit. How do you prioritize?

3. Reflect on the social determinants of health highlighted in this piece. What role did these factors play in the life of this patient?

—Aleena Paul

Being There

March 15, 2015

Corbin Pomeranz
Tulane University School of Medicine
Class of 2016

"IN ALL SERIOUSNESS," the attending physician says, "he can wear women's underwear to minimize the pain."

"Can he really?"

"Absolutely," replies the attending. "If we can't prescribe any pain medication, then tighter fitting clothing can help keep things from jostling about too much."

As we discuss alternative treatment options just outside his hospital room, I can hear our patient rolling around in his sterile white sheets, floundering to relieve the positional pain in his scrotum.

When he was diagnosed with stage IV hepatocellular carcinoma just days ago, his stage and prognosis made it seem like he had been battling the disease for years. I remember thinking someone with cancer this advanced must have noticed that *something* was wrong and would have sought medical attention months ago. In fact, his tumor was so large that upon initial inspection of his abdomen, what was thought to be impacted stool in his left lower quadrant was actually the cancer extending into his pelvis. The tumor was crushing the right side of his stomach, part of his duodenum, most of his ileum, all of his cecum, half of his transverse colon and completely obstructing his right testicular vein, causing his scrotum to swell to the size of a watermelon and become exquisitely painful. Every shift of his weight was accompanied by an audible high-pitched gasp as if he was struggling to undo a barbed-wire knot.

When you start your internal medicine rotation, your physician mentors express to you how many lives you'll touch and people you'll change for the better. No fresh third-year medical student is ever equipped to deal with the amount of personal anguish and pain one witnesses. My father is a physician and teaches medical students and residents. When I asked him what the hardest thing is for his new students to do, he looked at me, bowed his head, looked back up and said, "sitting beside suffering patients."

My attending starts up again.

"He wants to be discharged," he tells us, "and he wants to go back to work."

"What about the pain medications?" asks another med student.

"Unfortunately, because of his insurance and legal status, I can only write for a very limited supply," he replies. "After that, he'd have to wait till he's back in his home country."

"Wait, where is home?" I interject.

"El Salvador," replies the attending.

He had been working in northern Louisiana at a sugar cane factory for the last seven years. Every few months, he sent money back to his wife and five children in El Salvador. He said that he first noticed that he had been losing weight about eight months ago. He reported that it was about 20 to 30 pounds, which currently put him at around 100 pounds. The first symptom he experienced was a burning sensation that quivered down the lateral right side of his leg. Essentially, his lateral femoral cutaneous nerve was being compressed between his ilium and his inguinal ligament, creating a kind of carpal tunnel syndrome of the thigh. He had not thought much of it at the time and ascribed it to just being overworked. The disease silently progressed and about five months ago one of his coworkers noticed that he had "ixtelolohtli coztic," meaning "yellow eyes" in his native Nahuatl. Eventually, the abdominal pain started and one of his friends drove him to the hospital when he could not get out of bed. He said that he would lose his job if he did not go back to work. He just kept repeating, "pipiltzitzinti, pipiltzitzinti," which loosely translated into, "my children, my children."

It had been two days since we'd been able to reach a Nahuatl interpreter and since then we had been communicating in Spanish, which our patient spoke brokenly. Even so, the language barriers prevented our amorphous doctor-patient relationship from solidifying into genuine trust. We had another appointment scheduled for today at 10 p.m., seven hours from now.

"We need to explain to him how serious his situation is," says the attending. "I'm afraid the communication and cultural boundaries here are keeping him in the dark, which I am very uncomfortable with."

The attending would be doing the talking but I was afraid that I would feel like I did not belong there. I had heard about medical students who excelled during the first two years of medical school but when they started rotations, they could not stand being around sick people. I was terrified that I would be one of them.

Ten o'clock arrives with harrowing speed. We gather as a team in the patient's room about 15 minutes before the interpreter call. The attending kneels to the right of our patient, the receiver of the blue interpreter phone in his right hand, his left on the edge of our patient's bed. Our patient lies supine, his small 5-foot 4-inch frame ensconced in the large adjustable hospital mattress. Beads of sweat are forging visible moist trails from under his jet-black hair down his tanned sharply curved forehead and trailing laterally past his eyebrow. He is blinking a lot. As he puts the blue receiver up to his ear, a wave of intense pain hits him. He seizes, taking a deep breath in, his eyes opening wide towards the ceiling. The attending hurriedly captures our patient's hand in his and just holds it, sitting there silently for 30 seconds while our patient enters a visceral nightmare. When it's over, his muscles done reflexively contracting, our patient is aware of us again and he nods that he is ready to begin.

During my eight weeks on internal medicine, I witnessed some of the most remarkable instances of human physical findings, but they also came hand in hand with some of the most awful mortal circumstances one can be present for. As medical students, we are not always prepared for the ugly truths, but they are often where we can learn the most about our patients and ourselves. I learned that day how essential it is to be able to share in my patients' future triumphs as well as their losses. I learned that just being there can mean more than just "being there."

Questions

1. What experiences in your life, outside of the classroom, do you believe have prepared or equipped you as a future physician to bear witness to extreme anguish?

2. Put yourself in the place of the patient in this story. Honestly reflect on how you would want to be treated by the physician and medical students around you. What would you want them to say? What would you not want them to say and do?

3. No matter our different backgrounds, none of us are prepared for the tragedy that is human mortality. How will you process these experiences in a positive way? How can they help you mature?

—Eric Donahue

A Portrait of the Patient As an Old Man

March 19, 2015

Millin Sekhon
University of Miami Miller School of Medicine
Class of 2018

I LOOKED UP FROM my computer to motion the next patient in line and saw before me an elderly gentleman who resembled many of the other patients attending our health fair in Key West. Casually dressed: a white V-neck T-shirt and track pants. Hair: gray and wispy. Skin: tan and leathery from the sun. He was over six feet tall, with an athletic build for a man his age. It was approaching lunch hour and the line for my MED-IT station was dwindling.

"Sir, I can take you right over here," I gestured towards the seat across from my computer. He approached with what I interpreted as confusion, declining to sit.

"Are you getting your cholesterol checked today, sir?"

He seemed preoccupied and glanced around the room impatiently.

"I guess so — guess that's why I'm here, right?" He smiled tenuously and handed me his file.

But before I could ask whether he had been fasting, he broke in with, "A bear walks into a bar and says to the bartender, 'Gimme a beer.' The bartender replies, 'I don't give beer to bears in this bar.'"

Once he realized he had captured my attention, he dove into — essentially in one breath, as if diving into water — a long series of riddles, jokes and factoids, and once I had laughed at enough of his lines, he finally felt comfortable enough to sit down and introduce himself.

"My name is Patrick Goldenberg," he said, and tossed his driver's license nonchalantly across the table. He was slightly breathless from the aforementioned monologue, but when I spoke, he hung on to my every word, leaping at any chance to segue into a new story. He divulged, among other things, that his two siblings had been members of MENSA, and that both had committed suicide years ago. It became clear that he was rather brilliant — with a repertoire of endless dates and names at his fingertips — but he also possibly suffered from a mental illness. More or less modestly, he claimed to be 'no genius,' having taught sailing at Harvard and currently working as a professional card player. After several minutes I was able to gather that, according to him, this man had lived a very far-fetched life. But it wasn't so much his actual dialogue — fragmented stories, tangential recollections from childhood, movie recommendations — that resonated with me; it was the fervor with which he sought my attention. His tone conveyed, on the surface, a sense of entitled joie de vivre over which any elderly man could claim ownership. But closer inspection revealed a vague sense of gallows humor, and behind that, a jaded sense of reality. I was left with the impression that his tall tales, albeit eccentric, had not impinged upon his conception of the world. While I didn't perceive him as delusional, he was so focused on exuding this pseudo-savant persona that I began to feel like a tool for his own validation.

"Did you know that S-H-I-T is an acronym?" He sat facing my left, but as he asked, he turned towards me and put his hands on the table. I noticed his fingernails were quite dirty.

"In colonial times we would get our manure from England. How would they transport the manure, well, they would bring it over in boats. They would store the manure in the bottom of the boat, and what would happen? The manure would get wet, and the methane would cause explosions in the boat. That's no good. They decided that they needed to store the manure higher in the boat. *Higher in the boat.* So it wouldn't get wet. They put the manure in boxes high up in the boat. And what was printed on the cargo boxes? Ship. High. In. Transit. Ship high in transit." He nodded smugly and I expressed polite amazement, but in the back of my mind, wheels started turning: was he homeless? Were *any* of his stories true?

I now couldn't keep my eyes away from his dirty hands and fingernails, and I started questioning the last 30 minutes I had spent with Mr. Goldenberg. I was no longer so sure that he was in touch with reality — a reluctant dénouement on my end. Our interactions lasted a few minutes more and ended with Mr. Goldenberg adamantly suggesting I take his phone number, email address, and home address in case I ever needed a place to stay in Boston. He claimed that he would have asked me out to dinner that night, but he very strictly only dated women at least half his age. I had missed the mark by ten years. I printed the stickers for his cholesterol test and took my lunch break.

Weeks later, I still reflect on our meeting and wonder about the nature of reality when it comes to Mr. Goldenberg. I googled his address in Boston and found that it is the address of a sandwich shop. I searched his name in conjunction with "Harvard sailing professor" and found no results. But in a grand sense, does it really matter if he is real? Years from now I will most likely remember him just as he intended, a sharp old man replete with acronyms. And so I send him weekly emails and receive long messages in return, wrought with misspellings, often in all caps, and always brimming with random didacticisms. I store these pieces of advice like small gems. My most recent favorite is, "If a boy you like says lovingly or cutely 'what am I gonna do with you' it ain't a positive. He's saying you ain't got a good brain and he must make decisions for you."

A part of me knows that these emails are somewhat incoherent and logically should be taken with a grain of salt, but a small part of me wants to believe that there is profound meaning behind them. A moderate part of me wants to make an exegesis of Mr. Goldenberg's emails; perhaps he is the mortal embodiment of Zeus, veiled in semi-homeless garb to impart hidden truths. But a huge part of me knows that I tend to glean grand meanings from interactions that are only serendipitous at best, and I am wholly aware that life is not based on Homer's "The Odyssey."

Nonetheless, I will go to the ER to practice history-taking and leave raving about a homeless man who promised me he would quit drinking. I will carry his maxims with me to the grave, and I will be more touched by his affirmations than by any I could receive from my community preceptor. Why is that? Is it wise to assume more candor lies in members of subaltern groups? Regardless, there is a definite give-and-take in this unique relationship between doctors and patients. On the one hand, patients like Mr. Goldenberg want to be heard and, moreover, want to be seen in a certain way. But in regards to our own validation, is that not what we as medical students, as residents, as doctors, desire as well, from patients? All relationships lay claim to an extent of mothering, whether we see it or not. For the patient and the doctor, the reality is that both must believe in each other. And although I now assume that the majority of Mr. Goldenberg's emails are fabricated, I indulge him in the hopes that he finds solace in my faith in him. If for nothing but my own level of catharsis, *my* portrait of Mr. Goldenberg is all that matters. And in reality, I remain his pen-pal as an underwhelming attempt to repay him for what he said to me as he took back his driver's license, dirty fingernails and all.

As I got up to take my lunch break, he pointed to me and said, "This is a really good thing you're doing here. You."

Questions

1. It is often the role of the physician to discern truth from fiction. What are some ways that one can do this effectively? When is this distinction most important, and when is it not?

2. Describe an interaction you've had with a particularly colorful, memorable patient. What made this patient so memorable and what sort of positive or negative impression did he or she leave on you?

3. Imagine if the author had confronted the patient about some of his exaggerations or embellishments. How do you think the patient would have reacted, and how would this confrontation have impacted the patient-physician relationship?

4. Would you have established an email relationship with this patient? Why or why not?

—Yuli Zhu

Pansies, Rosemary and Rue

April 27, 2015

Erin Baumgartner
University of Louisville School of Medicine
Class of 2016

TRUTHFULLY, I PICK her name off the new patient list because it belongs to a woman, and several of our male patients have already come upstairs flagged for aggression. It is too early in the morning, and late in the week, and I haven't yet learned that female patients can be just as unpredictable as the men. I am in a hurry this morning, and I make the mistake of not skimming through her chart before I go in to see her. I don't know any more than the barebones: her name and her chief complaint upon admission.

I find her wandering the contours of her small room, which is set back in a mostly empty hallway. She is brandishing a toothbrush and a tube of toothpaste. Initially, I take this as a promising sign, but the incomprehensible muddle of words that tumbles out in response to my morning salutation dashes those hopes. The term that I will pen into the chart is "word salad." Taken aback, I pause, one foot bracing the door open. Almost immediately, I realize that there is no possible way I am going to get a meaningful interview this morning. Yet, I feel an obligation to at least give it a good effort. "How did you sleep last night?" The response is a crazy-quilt mish-mash of scenarios involving people who talk underwater, turkeys and flowers.

"...pansies, that's for thoughts..."

As I plaster my back to the wall behind me, she stands uncomfortably close, swaying inwards as though preparing to ask me a question. But she never quite manages to make the words line up in the correct order. I have never encountered someone so floridly psychotic before, and I am equal parts fascinated and horrified. I am unable to tell if she truly even registers my presence, if she knows where she is, or if I have simply been slotted into the cast of characters populating whatever strange drama is playing out behind her opaque brown eyes.

"...she chanted snatches of old tunes;

As one incapable of her own distress..."

I decide to call her Ophelia.

As is often the case with many of the patients with schizophrenia populating our inpatient ward, the psychiatry team can only assume that Ophelia is in the throes of her psychotic episode because she had stopped taking her medication. However, we will be unable to know for sure until she comes back to herself enough to tell us so. Her parents do not know, although they suspect that she has been neglecting to take her Risperdal. At first it does not appear as though there is going to be much improvement.

Over the course of the last few days of the week I watch her roam the common area, a bar of soap thrust out in front of her as though it is a compass. Perhaps she hopes it will help her map a route back to reality. Sometimes she totes around a rolled up towel, cradling it as though it is an infant. Other times she sidles up and stands on the fringes of our group during rounds, a something almost like a smile on her face. It is as though she thinks we are playing a game, and she is waiting to be picked for someone's team. I leave for the weekend without much hope. By the start of the next week however, the medication has begun to work its magic.

"...rosemary, that's for remembrance..."

On Monday, when I greet her with a "good morning," for the first time her eyes truly focus on mine. Although she is still prone to slipping into nonsensical wanderings, she is now capable of holding the better part of a conversation. There are still cracks in the healing façade of her mind, but the contrast between the two interviews is stunning. Especially since last week she had not even been capable of stringing two words together into a sentence. When I ask her if she has been taking her medications at home she gives me a guilty look, and shakes her head.

"There's rue for you, and here's some for me."

Before I met Ophelia, in a dim corner of my mind that I was always a little ashamed of, I thought of many of the inpatients on the psych ward as simply crazy. I had not yet made the connection between psychiatry and illness, but Ophelia was, perhaps, one of the most desperately ill patients that I have seen in my clinical rotations. She played a crucial role in changing how I thought of psychiatric patients. A sickness of the mind is as concrete and as damaging as any sickness of the body. It was only after this realization that I felt I really began to get the full measure of worth out of my psychiatry rotation. Rather than viewing my psychiatry rotation as an annoyance to be borne, I gained a deep respect for those doctors who stare into the shattered mirror of the human mind.

"...you must wear your rue with a difference..."

Questions

1. What pre-existing prejudices has practicing medicine dispelled for you? In turn, has your experience in medicine reinforced any biases you hold?

2. Can you think of a particular patient interaction that has made you aware of a prejudice or bias that you weren't previously aware you held? How did that interaction change the way you think?

3. The individuals we contextually label as patients are also humans capable of making their own decisions (with some exceptions, such as cases where there is a surrogate decision maker). What do we as physicians owe to patients who choose to disregard medical advice? In what ways can we help those whose choices do not line up with our medical opinion of what is best for them?

4. The author states that she "had not yet made the connection between psychiatry and illness." Do you think that society is moving toward or away from understanding this concept?

5. At one point in this narrative, the author is clearly distressed and possibly frightened because of the actions of her patients. What can we do to maintain a safe environment for ourselves as physicians as well as for our patients?

—Lindsey McDaniel

Communication and Miscommunication

Diversity, and Rhinos

September 24, 2012

Bianca Maria Stifani
Alpert Medical School of Brown University
Class of 2015

"ÚLTIMAMENTE ME HE sentido muy cansado," starts explaining Genaro. He has been feeling tired, but also weak, and unable to concentrate on things. Since he arrived in Providence a couple of years ago from the highlands of Guatemala, he has been doing hard work — manual labor like construction and carpeting, working long hours for little pay. "Se me olvidan las cosas," he continues. He has been forgetful, and has had trouble holding on to jobs. He is getting depressed because he doesn't know what is happening to him.

"Did he have any head trauma? Does he have trouble with his vision? Has he had thoughts of hurting himself or others? Does he have any other medical problems? When was the last time he saw a doctor?" Dr. Boulel asks me. And I translate into Spanish. That is the purpose of my presence at the free clinic today. But I already know that today there is more to be translated than just language. Genaro is confused by all these questions. He wants to know what is wrong with him, why won't the doctor just tell him? Surely there must be a pill he can take to go back to normal.

Dr. Boulel is from Syria. I know little about him but I think he has been in America for a long time, probably longer than Genaro and I combined. He knows Arabic, and his English, though heavily accented, is almost perfect. Genaro's language isn't Spanish, but Quiché. It's a Mayan language spoken by only one million people in the Guatemalan highlands. My knowledge of Spanish is supposed to make 'Latinos' feel comfortable. Dr. Boulel thinks Genaro feels at ease with me because of the Spanish, but doesn't know that Genaro barely knows it. Why should he, anyway? In Guatemala, it's the language of oppression. I am wondering if my presence is making things any better — does it help at all to attempt this translation, from one foreign language to another?

Dr. Boulel wants to do a MoCA. The Montreal Cognitive Assessment Test (MoCA) is a screening tool for rapid detection of cognitive impairment. The provider asks the patient a series of questions — some math, some language — and scores his answers on a scale of 0 to 30. A score of 26 and above is normal. Anything below that is abnormal. The test has been translated into 38 languages. Spanish is one, and so is Estonian (spoken by 1.1 million people in Estonia). But Quiché isn't. And what good would it be anyway, when neither of us speak it, and Genaro, most likely, doesn't read it? Dr. Boulel prints a Spanish copy of the test from the Internet.

The first question shows a bunch of letters and numbers randomly spread around a boxed area. An arrow points from number 1 to letter A and then to number 2. "Mira," I say. "Desde el numero uno se va hasta la letra A, y desde el numero dos ...Y así sigue ..." So it goes on. "Now you continue. What comes next?" Genaro stares at me. "After one comes two and then three and then four ... After A comes B and then C and then D ... No entiendo." I repeat the instructions but he meets me with the same blank stares. By now I am certain he must be thinking that I'm crazy. Now, as I write, I'm wondering — why is that we always think that by repeating the exact same thing many times, people will eventually understand us? As if the problem was theirs, as if they hadn't listened the first, second and third time, as if there was a switch they could suddenly turn on to understand us the fourth time? I wasn't explaining this well, and I didn't know how to. Dr. Boulel didn't know how to help. Maybe there was no way to help, and the question just didn't make any sense to begin with. If after 1 comes 2 and then 3, what do A and B have to do with it?

Genaro starts getting nervous because he realizes he is failing the test. Dr. Boulel is nervous because a) Don't I speak Spanish? Why doesn't the patient understand me? And b) Hasn't this guy been to school, or what? He decides we should move on to the next question.

"Draw a clock that shows 11:10." Genaro grabs the pen. "Once y diez?" he confirms. This time, he wants to get it right. Then he draws a rectangular digital clock display and carefully writes 11:10. He makes the numbers look like they would appear on a digital display with the one made out of two lines ... "No, I meant a clock like this one" and point to my own watch. He stares for a second then draws a circle. "I don't know these types of clocks" he says, and puts down the pen.

Dr. Boulel looks at me and sentences: "Okay, let's give him half the points."

Next come the animals. A lion, a rhinoceros and a camel are drawn on the page; they are staring at Genaro waiting for him to recognize and name them. The correct answer would be: "un león, un rinoceronte y un camello." Genaro stares at the animals and thinks. He thinks for a few minutes. Dr. Boulel and I get increasingly anxious. I am really wondering if these animals have ever been seen walking around the highlands of Guatemala, and cursing whoever thought it was a good idea to pick exotic, African animals to test the cognitive abilities of people all over the world. Why not a chicken, a dog and a cow?

In the end Genaro points at the lion and says "Creo que es un tigre." He thinks it's a tiger. Close enough. Dr. Boulel smiles, he will give him the point. Then Genaro points at the rhino and says in Spanish, "This ... Well, I don't know, but I think it's a cow." I can't resist and burst out laughing. It is completely unprofessional, I know, but too ironic to resist. There are few things the whole world has in common and one of those are cows. Maybe he's thinking that in America, where everything is different, cows' horns are in the middle of their faces instead of on top of their heads. I'm thinking that maybe in America, where everybody is different, they could have considered that some places don't have rhinos, but all places have cows.

Finally, he looks at the camel and gives up. Its neck is indeed too long for it to be a horse, plus it doesn't have a mane, its tail looks like a cow's, and what is up with that strange bump on its back?

I turn to Dr. Boulel and translate. Not just the language and the animal names but what I can imagine came behind them. I don't know much about Guatemala but I have been to Chiapas, Mexico, the region which borders Guatemala and shares many of its geographical features and ethnic groups. I think of the bright green hills and coffee plants and say "there are no rhinos, camels or lions in Guatemala. I don't think this reflects his cognitive ability."

"But didn't he see them in school?" the doctor asks. I am not sure about Syria, but I am guessing that there are no lions there either. Nor are there any in Italy, but both Dr. Boulel and I remember seeing pictures of these animals in grade school. But the schools I saw in Mayan communities in Chiapas were one-room shacks with a chalk board and children of all ages sharing a single bench. There were no picture books or computers. The students' notebooks were almost empty, and the few pages that weren't were used to practice the alphabet, and numbers. I didn't see a single rhinoceros.

I imagine that where Genaro grew up in Guatemala was somewhat similar to that. I explain this to Dr. Boulel. He gets it. Although he said earlier that this test "is supposed to be universal," he knows it's not, as nothing can be. He was just trying to be thorough, to quantify things, as we like to do in America. There is so much guessing going on when we try to understand where "people who are different from us" are coming from, what they are saying, what they want from us. Things like the MoCA are just a way to fool us into thinking we know something about somebody and their world, when really, we know nothing.

Genaro aces the next questions which are pure memory and math. I decide to change the words he has to memorize to things that make sense, picking "chicken" instead of "silk." Dr. Boulel is generous with his grading and Genaro gets a 27. Normal. Despite all of this he made it pretty clear to us that he is not cognitively impaired; if anyone in this room is, it is more likely to be one of us in white, asking absurd questions.

Dr. Boulel refers Genaro for an MRI and he is sent over to those who can help him schedule it. Although with no insurance, who knows if he will get one? I try to reassure him that his test was normal, and translate Dr. Boulel's explanations — "perhaps you are working too hard, perhaps you are feeling depressed, where is your family?" He wants to know what is wrong but we don't know. So he goes.

I haven't seen Genaro since but I have been thinking about him often, and about my role as an imperfect translator not only of languages but also of worlds. From Spanish to English, from Guatemala to Syria. I often think that because I myself am 'diverse,' because I am an immigrant, because I speak many languages, because I have traveled, I can provide better care than others could. But in this case, both Dr. Boulel and I, diverse as we are, failed Genaro. I can only guess, but we probably made him even more confused and distressed than he was when he came in. Will the MRI make any difference? Will it make him feel better? What if it comes out normal, as it most likely will?

Diversity means that people are actually all different from each other, not just from ourselves. So being diverse does not mean we will just 'get it.' There can be no manual for dealing with "diverse patients," be they "Latino" or "African," just like there can't be one for "White Americans." I do my best to take guesses and try to translate languages and worlds, but Genaro reminded me of the limits of language (and pictures), and gave me an important lesson in modesty.

Questions

1. Recall a time in which you worked with a patient of a different culture, language, socioeconomic status, religion or sexual orientation than you. What strategies helped to bridge these differences and lead to an effective, compassionate visit? What strategies did not work?

2. The author makes an interesting point in that the MoCA has been translated into Estonian (spoken by 1.1 million people) but not Quiche (spoken by 1 million people). Why do you think this is so? Do you think it is worth it to translate common medical tests like these into more languages, and why do you think they have not been yet?

3. The author notes that Genaro, being from the highlands of Guatemala, has probably never encountered a rhinoceros in his life or learning. Name some other examples of tests or scenarios that have inherent biases within them against people of certain cultures or backgrounds.

4. Have you ever worked with a medical interpreter in a clinic? What was the experience like and how did the presence of an interpreter affect the physician/patient dialogue and relationship? If not, what are some ways doctors and patients can communicate effectively without an interpreter?

—Yuli Zhu

Medicine, Meaning and Fluency: My Search for a Lingua Franca

October 12, 2012

Jocelyn Mary-Estelle Wilson
James H. Quillen College of Medicine
Class of 2013

W HAT I LOVE ABOUT medicine is that it is, in one sense, just another culture. It is a world of operational definitions. The ability to accurately describe an injury or procedure may be likened to gaining proficiency in a language. I remember learning French and pushing myself in order to express myself — to communicate. The desire to share ideas was so great that I had to learn; not just what to say, but *comment dire* — how to say it. We learn so much just as building blocks, to simply come to the table and be a part of the conversation. I am in pursuit of fluency. In practice, there is the need to speak to a colleague and the need to speak to a patient. One skill I felt that I was learning third year was the ability to communicate with my attending — to utilize doctor talk. On the other hand, lest we become too comfortable, there is the paramount need to communicate with the patient. "You're getting a Dobhoff because you're not stable enough for a PEG." Who understands that statement? The people I hang out with do (and secretly, I'm so impressed with myself that I'm finally putting some of this surgery stuff into my permanent memory). Deep sigh.

Recently, I watched a man improperly land with his foot inverted. He heard a snap or a pop and it immediately started to swell. Afterwards, he had good range of motion, could bear weight, had good dorsalis pedis and posterior tibialis pulses and had no bony tenderness. I told him a fracture was very unlikely. I also told him that I thought a rupture of a ligament or tendon was highly likely because of the things I described previously and the immediacy of the swelling he experienced. He looked at me and said, "When I hear the word 'rupture' I think of bombs blowing up." I thanked him for the feedback — yes, I used the word feedback. In my mind, many words presented themselves as options — avulsed, torn, and ripped. I think I said something about the grades of ankle sprains, the distinguishing factors between merely stretching a ligament, partially tearing it, and fully (I so want to say rupture again) tearing the ligament. Why does "rupture" seem like the perfect word to me, but such a horrible word to him? I've been in doctor land a long time I guess.

Is there a middle space?

Is there a medical language that has the precision of doctor language and the ubiquity of a pop song? The pop song reference was not chosen to suggest "annoyingly everywhere;" I chose it to suggest something readily accessible to the public and neatly fitting into the public's schema. It should be a language that uses tangible images so that we can make meaning together — with ease. I'm afraid such a language does not exist.

All of this turns my thoughts to the very definition of a professional. The term professional denotes a person who corners the market on a certain service or knowledge base. That is why there is credentialing. What if I wake up tomorrow and say, "I feel legal today. I'm going to open up a shop and take clients to defend their rights"? Hopefully only a small group would be fooled and quickly some governing body would stop me. There are exams and licensing bodies. All of this so that I can wave a paper and say I have a certain kind of knowledge — I've proved it by devoting myself to study, passing these tests. You can trust me to perform said skill. I have rights and responsibilities. But I digress.

There is a quote, attributed to Einstein, that says if you cannot describe it simply you do not understand it well enough.

I ardently desire this skill.

I still remember my cardiologist, Dr. Towne, taking a picture of a heart off his wall and marking on it with his pen to explain Wolf-Parkinson-White to the sixth grade version of me. I'm no electrophysiologist, but his explanation of atrioventricular reciprocating tachycardia still sticks with me. Instead of drowning in details, I want to have a command of pathophysiology, pharmacology, plan and prognosis. One day.

Questions

1. Give an example of a time when you encountered a mismatch between the language you used in a situation and the audience to whom it was directed. What are some techniques you can use to overcome this issue?

2. What are benefits to using esoteric or technical language? Pitfalls?

3. The author uses several examples of overly technical language. How do you instinctively react to her use of such language?

—Andy Kadlec

On Doctoring Etiquette

July 22, 2013

Qing Meng Zhang
Rush Medical College
Class of 2017

THE PATIENT WAS A woman in her mid-twenties recently diagnosed with lupus. She was clearly anxious about her prognosis and treatment. The rheumatologist I was shadowing that day entered the room, made some casual conversation intermingled with medical questions, and proceeded with the physical exam. She was attentive to the patient's needs and accommodating with her questions. The rheumatologist's confidence, compassion and ability to sooth the patient's worries made a lasting impression on me. During the brief 15 minute encounter, she not only listened to what the patient had to say, answered every question she had, and communicated her thoughts clearly, but she also made small talk, which made the visit more like a casual encounter with an acquaintance and less like a doctor's appointment.

Bedside manner and customer service skills have been climbing up the ladder of importance in health care and physicianship. In Western culture in particular, patient satisfaction and customer service are highly valued because they are great marketing strategies. From restaurants to car dealerships, businesses rely on customers' satisfaction and devotion. Hospitals, likewise, are businesses that need an influx of customers and depend on profits. Many websites, such as vitals.com and healthgrades.com, provide physician information to the public along with reviews of physicians by patients. This provides patients with the transparency required to make informed decisions on choosing the right physician.

Physicians are not only healers that alleviate physical discomfort. They also act as social workers and psychiatrists to care for the mental health and emotional states of their patients. I have seen very intelligent physicians being turned away by patients due to their subpar bedside manner. Clinical competency is a must, but qualities like clear and effective communication, ability to connect with other people on an emotional level, and negotiation skills have become equally important. Studies have shown that patients are less likely to sue physicians with better bedside manner than those with inadequate bedside manner when clinical competency is equal.

However, this is not to say that customer service should actually replace clinical competency. After all, would you rather be seen by a physician of great intelligence and expertise but mediocre bedside manner, or by an extremely charismatic physician with limited experience? The first and foremost duty of any physician is to ease patients' pain and discomfort, and this is usually performed best with sufficient knowledge. A great physician is someone who can incorporate both qualities with every patient.

Despite the glamour and importance of bedside manner, it is easier said than done. For example, look at our day-to-day conversations with friends and families. We often feel the urge to interrupt another person's sentence because we feel strongly about a point they just made, or our body language may give away some of the feelings we prefer to hide. Similarly, throughout a visit, the physician needs to attentively listen to the patient's history while appearing sympathetic, be aware of any body language, and yet still formulate a clinical plan. Many physicians are even able to conduct a full physical exam at the same time. Truly, this takes multitasking to a whole new level.

Recognizing the importance of exhibiting interpersonal skills among physicians and teaching doctoring etiquette to medical students, most medical schools in the United States have included "Physicianship", "The Art of Medicine", or "Preceptorship" in the first-year curriculum. As a result, medical students are able to shadow physicians interacting with patients early in their training so that they not only learn and practice obtaining a solid patient history and conducting physical exams, but are also ingrained with the do's and don'ts in medical settings.

Clearly, all the necessary qualities of excellent physicians are not easily obtained. It requires dedication and compassion, as well as years of experience and practice. Hopefully, one day we may all reach our goal of being fully competent, compassionate and caring physicians.

Questions

1. The author writes: "Clearly, all the necessary qualities of excellent physicians are not easily obtained." Do you feel that you receive sufficient instruction and mentoring on all of the necessary qualities of excellent doctoring? Do you think bedside manner is innate, or can it be learned?

2. Have you encountered physicians who showcase examples of subpar bedside manner? If so, what actions stuck out to you the most?

3. The author references websites where patients can leave reviews of physicians. Do you think these websites play a significant role in helping patients choose physicians? What should physicians do if they receive negative reviews?

4. What qualities do you want of your personal physician? What qualities do you want of the physician of your significant other? Your friends? Your family? Should you think about these qualities when evaluating your own bedside manner?

—Melanie Watt

A Patient in Denial: Is the System at Fault?

November 7, 2014

Ola Hadaya
Wayne State University School of Medicine
Class of 2016

I'VE COME TO REALIZE having an automatic word filter is one of my greatest blessings. It becomes quite useful when, in the middle of rounds, a patient's single, monosyllabic response inspires such a flurry of mismatched curse words that only a properly formed filter can save my dignity. What exactly did this patient say that stunned me so violently?

My attending had asked him a straightforward, albeit grim, question. "Do you know you have cancer?"

The patient had gawked at her, his head slightly reeled back, eyes wide. "No."

His response wouldn't have shocked me had he not been diagnosed with prostate cancer seven years ago, had he not had multiple prostate biopsies demonstrating super high Gleason scores, had he not continued following up with his primary care physician, who took routine PSA measurements year after year. When we think of health care and people "falling through the cracks," we nod our heads solemnly at the data, the people who didn't follow up in clinic and ended up worse than before, the poor who couldn't afford insurance and so stayed away until they couldn't tough it out anymore. You know. *Those* people.

But this patient wasn't one of those statistics. He had kept his appointments, had done the recommended testing — how could he not have known he had cancer? What kind of health care system exists where a patient gets continuous specialized tests without understanding their grave meaning?

Surely, I thought as I returned to my base pod, surely something somewhere in the system failed him. Doing procedures for seven years without knowing why — is this what poor health literacy was? Had all his doctors used so much jargon he couldn't understand?

No, that explanation seemed too simple. Jargon or not, the word cancer is universally known and feared.

Perhaps it was the severity of his disease he did not understand. Denial could have played a role, too, but when your PSA grows year by year, when your cancer reaches a Gleason score of nine, it would seem to me denial would have one hell of a job maintaining ignorance. It's not entirely farfetched that an uneducated man with cancer, having not undergone any dramatic chemotherapy or gory surgery or other TV drama ready procedure, could have possibly underestimated the scale of his illness. And even if he *were* in pure denial of his aggressive cancer, shouldn't the health care system have picked up on this and consulted psychiatry or a therapist or someone to help re-explain his situation to him?

I spent many hours thinking about this case. Had the health care system failed this man, who was either in obvious denial of his illness or genuinely uninformed about the severity of his cancer? Or had his PCP and other players in the field tried their best to educate him but failed? I don't think I'll ever get a nice, clear answer. I'd have a better chance — and a bigger waistline — winning a chocolate statue of myself. All I can say for sure is that after our team treated him for dehydration, malnutrition, and other issues that arose from his metastatic cancer, our patient asserted he would see the appropriate doctors for his follow up.

Judging by his recent medical records, he did.

Somehow, his inpatient stay with us got through to him regarding the gravity of his illness, but I can't help but wonder: was it too late? Yes, his condition has improved, and he's gained some weight, putting meat on his cachectic frame, but let's face it: he has metastatic prostate cancer. Had he known exactly what his rising PSA levels had meant, would he have elected to have his prostate removed, thus avoiding the death sentence he has now?

The health system helped him in the beginning by providing him with a diagnosis and at the end by treating the impacts of his illness, but to me, perhaps due to my naïveté in believing denial can't be the sole explanation for this story, we let him down in the middle of his journey, where he should have had our support and attention most, where he could have healed.

Or I could be wrong.

Maybe my more cynical residents are right. Maybe he was in seven years of denial, and either no one picked up on it or couldn't get through to him. I guess all I can really say about the impact of the health care system on this particular patient is that it was 100 percent certainly ambiguous.

And that's terrifying.

Believing the system *could* have had a hand in all these complications, that a patient with a grave disease *could* have not understood the severity of his disease, that a patient *could* have been clueless as to the significance of his tests, that a life saving procedure *could* have been passed up due to a patient's poor medical knowledge, that signs of denial *could* have been missed by professionals who regularly saw their patient — I'll say it again. *Terrifying.* None of these "coulds" should exist, and yet they do.

People love asking and reflecting on how the health care system plays a role in the outcome of patients. Truth is, for this poor man, with the information I have, the only information I'll probably ever have, I don't know. But with all the "coulds" that come to mind, does that even matter?

Questions

1. For those who "fall through the cracks" due to poverty or misfortune, is it our responsibility as future physicians to assure they receive all the care needed? Is it society's responsibility? The government's?

2. In your medical training and future career you will encounter "those people." Stereotypes aside, what level of responsibility do you feel that the physician must hold to assure such patients are not lost to their ignorance, denial or just blatant misunderstanding? At what level must we educate and confirm their understanding?

3. The limits of the current health care system are evident to us. The "coulds" that the author alludes to are terrifying. What would you like to see changed in the system to combat these unfortunate situations? What do you believe your role should be in that change? What do you believe the role of the collective should be?

—Eric Donahue

Clinical Culture Shock: Low Health Literacy as a Barrier to Effective Communication

November 11, 2014

Lindsey McDaniel
University of Kansas School of Medicine – Wichita
Class of 2016

O N A SATURDAY MORNING at one of our local safety net clinics, where third-year medical students see patients independently and then present to the supervising attending, a man in his 60s arrived to talk about some lab results he had received and what they meant. This man, Mr. S, had many medical problems, including hypertension, COPD, chronic kidney disease and newly diagnosed diabetes. He came to the office that day wanting to know why he had several abnormal values on his most recent lab work. Mr. S clearly wanted to take care of his own health as best he could, but like many patients he had very low health literacy. Confounding this situation was the advice of his neighbor, a chemist, who informed him he needed several more tests done, further confusing Mr. S.

"Why am I anemic? What does it mean that I have high parathyroid hormone? My neighbor told me that y'all need to do these tests here," he told me, pointing to the hand-written words 'transferrin' and 'thyroid panel' on his lab results sheet. Since this was the first time I had encountered this patient, his lab results were a bit of a conundrum to me at first as well. When I looked at his whole picture and the other medical conditions he had while presenting to my attending, his lab results made more sense. Mr. S had chronic kidney disease, which easily explains both of the abnormal results; his kidneys weren't secreting enough erythropoietin to stimulate sufficient red cell growth, and they also weren't reabsorbing enough calcium and activating enough vitamin D to satisfy the sensitive parathyroid glands.

Explaining this to a man with low health literacy was simultaneously simple and challenging.

"Your kidneys aren't working as well as we would like, so we want you to see a nephrologist, a kidney specialist, who can help you manage that better," my attending explained when we saw the patient together. Mr. S accepted

218

that, but when I went back to give him his paperwork, he had a little more to say when I asked him if he was satisfied with the answers we had given him. He thought he understood our explanation well enough, but he wondered what could he have done to have prevented this. He felt neglected by the specialists he had seen in the past, both because of his uninsured status and because he hadn't understood their explanation of his condition well. He was concerned that he would be written off again. This time, the only care I could provide was to listen and reassure.

Overall, I sent Mr. S home feeling like our health care team hadn't helped him all that much. He was a very pleasant, talkative gentleman who clearly wanted to have a voice in his own care. He seemed satisfied for now, but I wasn't. I had listened to his concerns and tried to translate the medicalese I have been learning for the past two and a half years into something he could understand. But I didn't feel like I had done a very good job. I realized then how important it is to find a way to help people of all educational levels understand enough to be an active player in their own health care, and how difficult it can be to find the right words for each patient. I hope that the more I talk with patients, the better I will become at doing this.

So many people, myself included, say that we want to go to medical school to help people. One of the hardest realizations to make is that we can't always help people in the grand ways we once pictured. Sometimes all we can do is listen and make sure that the patient feels heard and respected. Sometimes we have a medical intervention that will improve that person's life to some degree. Sometimes we have a medication that will make it worse for a while in hopes of making it better in the long term. Sometimes we see well people and try to help them stay well. The important thing is that we never lose the desire to help and to keep trying to help in the face of encounters that feel futile or patients who can't always help themselves.

Questions

1. Think of a patient interaction in which low health literacy played a role. What steps did you take to help your patient?

2. In what ways can physicians and health care organizations address low health literacy among their patients? How do you approach a patient who might be making an unsound medical decision because of his or her low health literacy?

3. How do we as providers distinguish between "low health literacy" among our patients and our use of medical terminology or jargon that is unfamiliar to our patients?

—Aleena Paul

Talking Dirty

December 2, 2014

Mariya Cherneykina
Temple University School of Medicine
Class of 2017

B ARELY INTO MY second year of medical school, I already have a reputation — I love asking the uncomfortable stuff. Social history, sex, drugs,
alcohol, I want to know it all. At first, it was just because that section randomly fell on me during small group sessions or standardized patient encounters. Then, I began to volunteer, or be volunteered. "Mariya loves the
dirt," my classmates say.

Without saying, I always approach this section of the interview with
the finest nuance of word, a neutral demeanor and utmost professionalism.
However, my propensity toward asking these questions and knowing their
answers highlighted a palpable sense of curiosity that my classmates and
preceptors could feel. A long-time friend and dental student proposed that
it's the housewife in me — seeking something juicy and novel in the lives of
others to stir up the occasional banality of my own existence. Maybe, but to
her fortune (or perhaps misfortune), her patients' mouths are far too occupied to talk, so I did not find her observation to be entirely objective.

Then, I thought about conversations with my father, who as a former
medical examiner, saw the most atrocious and horrific ends to people's lives.
I often asked how he could remember his experiences without dwelling on
the disturbing memories of these events, how he never became consumed
with their suffering or the sheer effects of seeing such unsettling things. Instead, with his impeccable and jovial humor he could recount cases that
would land most people in psychotherapy. His answer was that he always
saw the bodies as objects of his work, always with an emotional distance.
For him, practice was all science; for me, practice is all feelings. I guess
that's why he's a pathologist and I spent four years studying psychology.

My curiosity for those uncomfortable questions is partly about getting
closer to the patient emotionally. However, it's not just in being able to elicit

a relationship of comfort and trust, but also in helping *me* better care for my patients. Patients are not just biological machines with errors to fix. After all, radiating chest pain and cough with sputum is not what makes someone a human being. What makes them human is that they are flawed, fallible and subject to a vast range of emotions. In the long run, isn't that what we're here to do? To heal pains of the human experience?

My asking of these questions in itself is part of the healing process for my patients. Without doubt, the sheer catharsis of sharing personal troubles with an unbiased party is therapeutic alone. At the same time, by becoming curious about your patients, you open the door to address their heroin use, impotence, unsafe living conditions or other issues too crippling to offer up voluntarily. It allows you to offer them at least the hope of someone understanding and being able to help. By asking these questions you find out that the noncompliant patient is terrified of medications because she accidentally overmedicated and killed her infant son, or that the "frequent flyer" is ailing from a broken heart. Most importantly for me, the "dirt" breaks the coldness of the sterile medical environment and impassions me to heal these people, not as objects of my work, but as humans.

Questions

1. What were your expectations when you read the title of this piece, and how do they compare with your feelings after reading it?

2. What techniques do you use to delve into sensitive matters with patients?

3. Have you ever felt like you've lost the human connection when talking to patients? If so, what did you do to regain it?

—Sasha Yakhkind

Lost in Translation

December 15, 2014

Katharine Caldwell
University of New Mexico School of Medicine
Class of 2016

I N THE REST OF the house, the noise of the party is deafening: the clink of glasses, the sizzle of burgers on the grill, the excited cries of relatives reunited after long absences. But in the bright light of the kitchen, Mark is talking to me without sound. He presses his right hand over his left then moves up its length, separating his thumb from the rest of his fingers as he goes replicating the open and shut motions of a jaw. "This is the sign for cancer," he says.

"Ooh, creepy," I cringe. "I didn't know ASL was so morbid."

"Exactly," Mark agrees, punctuating this with open hands. Mark is an American Sign Language interpreter and, even when not working, a little bit of gesticulation is to be expected when he speaks. "So that's why her son got mad at me."

Mark has been explaining to me how he had been translating for a client at her doctor's appointment and had been given the unfortunate task of delivering the news that this woman had cancer. When he'd done this, using the sign for cancer that he had just demonstrated to me, the woman's son had become very agitated and snapped at him.

"I don't think I would have liked the picture of something eating my mother either, to be perfectly honest. So what did you do? Spell it out?" I ask. I'm certainly showing my ignorance of ASL here, but I'm genuinely curious.

"I used a couple of other signs for the same idea." He says and his fingers unconsciously form them in the space between us. I'm not sure he realizes he's done it, and they flash by so quickly I'm not able to gather what they mimic.

"The metaphor of it is so different from English. Much more graphic. I guess that's the nature of a visual language, but I'd just never thought about it."

"It makes translating very..." he pauses, searching for the word. He finally settles on "strange," but doesn't seem quite content with it, and he quickly revises it to "challenging."

"You have to think about a thousand different things. I'm always having to think about what's being said and how that translates into sign, but also the way it was said and how to convey that. Sometimes I have to think about the setting — some of the ASL gestures are just more graphic and might not be appropriate in certain settings. I dance around a lot of things to fit the tone of the conversation."

"Like saying 'passed away' instead of 'died?'"

"Exactly. I just end up changing a lot of the words so I keep the intention and the meaning of the speaker because I can't always hold 100 percent to the words. Not everything translates."

I laugh. I tell Mark that is a feeling I am very familiar with. Although I'm sure that translating from one spoken language to another is nothing like the challenge presented by translating a spoken language to a signed one, I am familiar with the feeling of confusion at exactly how to translate the untranslatable. I tell Mark the danger of ever letting anyone at a hospital know that you speak another language. As a medical student, the second a doctor I'm working with notices me speaking with a patient in Spanish, I quickly find that I'm being grabbed and asked to translate in every situation that arises — many beyond my level.

I'm constantly turning people down when they ask me to translate. I don't have the skill to communicate the results of the MRI with this patient because I'm not sure how to say "adrenal gland" or "not concerning for malignancy." I don't have the comfort level to ask a patient very detailed questions about his or her medical history, where one error — one transposed word — could change a treatment plan.

But often times I do step up and try to help physicians communicate with Spanish-speaking patients. I often work as a stop-gap measure until a translator arrives in emergency situations, or I step in when I realize an attending is going to do that thing where you just speak very slow English to a non-English speaking person in hopes that they'll somehow be able to understand just by decreasing the velocity of the words thrown at them. I hate when people do that. I don't speak Chinese. I will not speak Chinese no matter how slowly you speak it to me. I can't learn the language in the pauses between your words.

When I do step in and translate, or even when I step in to have a primary bilingual encounter with a patient, I always do so with a disclaimer to the patient that my Spanish isn't perfect, but I'm going to try and if they ever are confused by what I'm saying or feel I'm misunderstanding them, they should stop me and we will wait for the translator. I often repeat back to patients what I think they've said to me to ensure I've gotten the right message.

I am a very cautious translator.

What always fascinates me is how quickly I find myself editing what's said. I find myself unable to grab for the exact translated word in Spanish, so I walk around what was said in English using two or four or six words to get there. Sometimes words are traded out for synonyms. Idioms are lost. It's what I can do. This is likely most often a failing of my own language skills, but sometimes the result of an idea or phrasing that simply does not exist in one language or the other.

I try to be as faithful as possible to the intention of what was said, even when the words themselves don't always seem to come out identical.

But no matter how much double checking I do, how simple the encounter, serving as the translator, the go-between, always makes me nervous.

How much did I lose?

How much slipped past me unsaid?

Did I fail to really express the doctor's concern? Did that really come across as a joke?

Did I fail to communicate the patient's fear, their anxiety?

Was I wrong to have switched out the patient's choice of "tube" for the more medical "drain" when she was speaking?

How much is lost on my lips?

All of medicine is a translation game because medicine itself speaks a language that often bears little resemblance to English, with most of its being composed of a bastardized Latin or Greek. Half of its thoughts are shortened into acronyms or nicknames, and a portion of its terms are archaic references to things long since forgotten. We spin together sentences full of lab values and statistics and the names of tests that we don't even know what all the letters stand for anymore.

How can you expect someone who speaks a traditional American-idiom to follow a conversation filled with words like "hyperplastic," "myeloma" and "choledocholithiasis?" Three years into my medical training and sometimes the details, the nuances of these conversations, slip past me. I should keep a list of the strange abbreviations or words I've looked up. Surgery seems especially bad at this, just squishing together all the words we want to say into one big mess and adding a suffix: pancreatoduodenectomy, esophagogastroduodenoscopy, choledochojejunostomy.

Sometimes, I've wondered if doctors use this language to keep themselves at arm's distance from the patient when things are uncertain or terrifying. Is medical jargon some sort of clinical coat that we wear, not only to distance ourselves from the reality of suffering all around us, but also to evade the painful realities of medicine?

Certainly medicine is an imperfect and unpredictable science. Perhaps we use medical jargon to hedge our bets. We've all seen ninety-year-olds come back from multi-organ failure while nine-year-olds die on the table with nothing more than acute appendicitis. We've seen poly-trauma victims recover completely normal function and simple fractures lead to lifetimes of disability and pain. We've seen non-treatable, 90 percent dead-in-a-year cancers turn to no evidence of disease, while 99 percent survival at five years end up in the one percent. We've seen the amazing turnarounds, the long shot winners, and the miracles. But we've also seen the nasty shocks, the one in a million, and the impossible heartbreaks.

We say "the CT was concerning for distant metastasis" instead of "your cancer will kill you before Christmas." We say "the speed of resuscitation was inadequate and it appears your loved one no longer has higher cortical functioning" instead of "your husband bled out too quickly. We couldn't stop it, and now he's dead. His body just doesn't know that his brain isn't functioning anymore."

Do we simply talk this way because the cool, clinical language of science is the one we have grown so accustomed to speaking that we forget many people are not as fluent as we are? We forget that many people have barely enough competency to know when to nod along.

Do we say these things because we're hoping that what we know to be true is wrong? We're hoping for the miracles, knowing they won't come, but not wanting to take that hope away from those people who still believe in them.

Do we say these things because if we dared to say "will be dead," "will not recover" or "permanent pain" it might burn us to sit so close to the fire of day-to-day suffering?

Or do we simply say it because we have not been taught the ability to translate our medical language into English? We are not certified translators; we are human beings with some bilingual proficiency trying to step around the sentences, and trying to hold onto the concepts and feelings. And sometimes we fail.

It's probably, on any given day, any or all of these things.

—

Eddy used to listen to Jimi Hendrix or the Grateful Dead. He's probably got Jefferson Airplane vinyls hidden in the dusty corner of some closet in his house. Now, even well past his bell-bottom pants and flowered shirts, he still retains some of that same vibe. I might walk in one morning and have him hand me a flower and tell me about how nuclear disarmament is the most important political issue. After free love, of course.

Eddy was admitted to the hospital for emergency surgery and it was during that emergency that he was first told he had end-stage cancer. Up until that point he'd been feeling fine, maybe a little bit more tired than usual, but his wife had been sick recently and it was probably because of that.

I remember the first time I saw him in the emergency department. He was wearing the same look as a student who thought he had sat down in his English class only to find himself in Japanese 201. He looked so overwhelmed, lost, and very small in that bed. He was thin, certainly the result of the all those years of cancer left festering deep inside his body unknown to him. But the smallness was greater than that, as though the cancer had eaten away more than just tissue, but part of his substance.

I think of Mark in the kitchen moving his hand up his arm.

Eddy's ribs poked through his chest, his sternum dipped slightly. Hands, chest, face: pale. That his H&H (blood numbers — there I am, speaking medicine) would show severe anemia was a surprise to no one. Every time I see him, I feel helpless. One of my attendings on surgery likes to say "a chance to cut, a chance to cure."

Here there is only a chance to cut.

Over the course of the next couple of days, Eddy underwent a very long series of surgeries. After one of many, we go see him on rounds.

My resident flicks the light on without warning, without introduction. No "hello," no "good morning," just bright lights and "surgery team here." He does the quick incision checks required: incisions clean, dry, intact, wound edge non-erythematous without drainage.

Just as we're about to step out, my resident drops that someone will be coming by today to take him for the CT.

"What CT?" Eddy asks. He's slightly slow to speak. My resident had almost made it to the door by the time the question leaves his lips.

"To see if the cancer has any more sites in your liver."

"But I thought you took that one out when you did the surgery."

"No, we just biopsied one of them. We're not going to remove them." My resident says and then he hits the door.

I can see it on Eddy's face. He has more questions. He hasn't understood even though it's been said to him half a dozen times in strange, clinical sentences. The fact that his cancer has metastasized to his liver means he's stage four, it means he's going to die, it means there's not much more to do now, maybe some palliative treatment, but no chance of cure anymore. I know I've heard a dozen different people in a dozen different white coats tell him these things, but it was all in these unclear, roundabout ways.

I should say something, I should call my resident back. But he's already on the phone to the operating room; first case is already asleep in the room. He's gone. He's already half scrubbed.

But I say nothing.

Stupid.

—

"What would you do?" Eddy asks me the next time I go by to see him, this time alone. "Why should I even bother? This has been hard enough on my wife figuring out that I have cancer. If she knew that it was in my liver too I think it would kill her. I don't think she could handle it. Would you have the CT? I don't know if I want to know. Does that make sense?" I'm not sure he's talking to me or just to himself or to the universe, but then he looks at me with his eyes large in their hollow sockets and waits for an answer.

And oh God, I wish that he hadn't asked. I don't know what I'm supposed to say. Should I tell him what I know about the numbers and the survival rates? Should I tell him that no matter what the CT shows, he's not going to ever get to be a cancer survivor? Should I do what everyone else has done and dodge the question with more numbers, more big words, so as to not have to be the one to hand him the finality of his diagnosis? Should I escape the conversation with an answer that he will be unable to translate?

I start to. I start to give him the same information he's been handed a dozen times, but the words die in my mouth. That's not what he needs.

Should I just tell him the truth — that if it were me, I'd check myself out of the hospital right now, fly to the Caribbean and spend the last six months of my life on the beach?

That's not what he needs either. This isn't about me. He just needs a translator. Someone to translate his emotions into a medical response that the doctors will understand. He needs someone to translate his "I need time to think about this" into medical speak.

"You don't have to have it done if you don't want to," I say, finally. "It's okay if you need to think about what you want. It's okay if you tell them that. They will understand. They were just trying to expedite things for you by having it done now, but they can always do it outpatient after you get discharged."

He says nothing for a long time. He looks up at the ceiling above him, a ceiling he must have been staring at for the last several days. I'm sure he is incredibly familiar with the place where the ceiling meets the lights, the place the paint is cracked. He's memorized the details of it all but this time I think he's looking for the answers. I don't think he'll find them.

"Thank you." He says at last and turns back to look at me. It's a soft, genuine "thank you." One that curls up the corners of his lips as it leaves them behind.

I'm certain I've said the wrong things, just as I do in Spanish. I'm certain I've failed to communicate appropriately what I mean to say, but I hope that he's heard the intention in there somewhere and that it's a comfort to him for me to speak the same language he speaks in lieu of the medicine he's heard too often.

—

Medicine permeates our speech. Being a doctor is much like being bilingual in a country that speaks predominantly a language that is different than the one you speak at home. You go to work and speak Medicine. You text it to your colleagues. You converse in it while you wait in line for coffee. You write it. You dictate in it. Then you come home, switch back to normal English, and your partner stops you halfway through a sentence because you've lost him or her down the rabbit hole of shortened words. You send an email to your mother with "s/p" and "2/2" found in the body and she thinks they're typos.

We speak Medicine and we do it so easily, so quickly, and so completely that we fail to recognize that someone else might have trouble understanding the tangled idiom of our sentences.

What I'm learning in the third year of medical school is that as doctors we have to wear a very large number of coats. Sometimes we're healers, sometimes counselors, sometimes teachers and sometimes translators. And sometimes we're especially bad at wearing that last coat enough. I don't know whether we just have to learn by experience, or this is something that we should be teaching our doctors to do.

I don't know if it's something I'll ever be good at it, or if I will always feel like I do when I try to translate to and from Spanish: like there's a chance I'm missing something, like there's a chance something is being left on my lips.

I do know that I must always strive to ensure the meaning is heard and the intention understood even when the words themselves are clumsy. Because Mark is right: not everything translates.

Questions

1. Consider the author's statement: "doctors use this language to keep themselves at arm's distance from the patient when things are uncertain or terrifying." Is there truth to this statement? Do we use medical language as a shield?

2. How can we provide humanistic care to our patients in situations where there is a communication barrier?

3. Have you been part of a patient encounter where the conversation did not "translate"?

4. Have you worked with a resident who treated a patient like the surgical resident treated Eddy in this narrative? How did you feel about the resident's behavior? What do you think about the author's initial reaction? Would you react any differently?

5. How did the author show respect for her patient Eddy by returning to discuss the CT scan?

—Aleena Paul

View From the Other Side

January 3, 2015

Jimmy Yan
Schulich School of Medicine & Dentistry
Class of 2015

"HE ALWAYS DOES THIS, it's unbelievable!"

My preceptor's voice was unmistakable. We had just finished our first case and I had momentarily left to get some coffee.

"This is getting unacceptable, someone needs to bring this up to the board!"

I had never seen him so worked up after having worked with him over the course of the week. Whatever this issue was, it clearly had been festering for while. From the sounds of it, the person in question has had a habit of this particular behavior.

"I agree, he keeps getting away with it and figures someone else will be there to pick up the slack," said another anesthesiologist.

"It's a typical surgeon's mentality, they all just want to operate and then not deal with patients afterwards," chimed in a nurse who was on her break.

"Whoa, *I* operate *and* see my patients plenty," said one of the orthopedic surgeons. "Don't lump us all into the same group here."

It was getting a bit uncomfortable in the staff room, especially for a visiting medical student who had only been here for a week.

"I think I'll go check on our next patient," my voice rasped. This was a bit of a lie as I knew the next patient was not in the pre-op room; I just needed a parachute and, in turn, I hurried out.

As the day continued, I heard more and more snippets of what was happening. Putting all the parts together, it seemed like the commotion was about a particular surgeon who allegedly went ahead and booked a patient for an operation at the end of the day, even calling to tell that patient to come down to the hospital without informing anyone else ahead of time. People were frustrated with having to work longer, rescheduling other cases on the trauma list and just the blatant disregard for process.

At the end of the day the surgery did occur but the surgeon in question did have a reason for his actions: his patient was riddled with widespread metastatic colon cancer. The patient and his family had different views on how to move forward on treatment, with the family wishing for palliation while the patient was still hoping for a cure. Finally, this surgeon agreed to conduct an exploratory laparotomy on the patient to see if there was any portion he could possibly resect or at least definitively ascertain the prognosis. Unfortunately, there was nothing to be done because the abdomen was riddled with tumor. Following the operation, the surgeon phoned in the family and stayed near the patient's bay until the patient and the family was ready to hear the news.

This experience reinforced the notion to me that there's always more than one side of an experience in medicine. It's easy to craft and follow stories that have clear "heroes" and "villains" but when does reality ever exist in such distinct dichotomies? All too often, easy short cuts are applied in the hospital setting which lead to labeling people, for example the "cold" surgeon or the "whiny" patient. One of the most important reasons to further explore the narratives in medicine is that doing so breaks past initial labels and allows us to better understand patients, how their experiences have shaped them and where they see themselves in our care.

Questions

1. Considering the title, what "sides" exist in the story? In contemporary medical culture? To which side does the medical student belong?

2. Were the actions of the surgeon justified? As physicians, are there times when we are justified in deviating from a standard of care, or does the standard of care serve a critical role in enabling us to provide the best care?

3. Have you witnessed a deviation from standard of care? Is that what is happening in this narrative, or is the surgeon providing a different kind of care for this patient?

4. The orthopedic surgeon in the story retorts, "Don't lump us all into the same group here." Can you think of certain traits that you typically associate with the different medical specialties? Do you think these stereotypes are accurate?

—Ileana Horattas

Doctoring: Who Is It Really For?

February 10, 2015

Nita Chen
Albany Medical College
Class of 2017

IN CHINESE, THE TERM for doctor is *yi sheng*, which roughly translates into "medicate to life." From this interpretation, the mission of a physician is to restore livelihood to patients, whether in the literal or in the metaphorical "wholesomeness of life" sense. While this may seem intuitive, the ingredients of "quality of life" and "satisfactory care" are much less clear and much more complex.

It is natural for us, as students of logic and problem solving, to treat medicine as a series of causes and effects. Much of our training pushes us to do our best to match patient presentation with classical textbook diagnoses. If there was an ultimate handbook of all the possible combinations of diseases and sufferings, it would solve much of our frustrations.

But in so many ways, this analytical, black-and-white method of perception constitutes a small iceberg chip among the multiple tenets of being a competent physician. Despite our movement away from overbearing paternalism with modern medicine, we still often believe we know what's best for our patients. It is so easy for us to reason through the "obvious" best course of action, that we often forget the unique and complex social context that every patient brings besides their presenting symptoms.

These thoughts began to plume in my mind when I received a phone call from my unhappy mother. She had just returned from an unpleasant visit to her endocrinologist. Earlier this year around March, she had first met with the endocrinologist, and she felt comfortable with his patience and open attitude. However, this time, she returned from the office feeling threatened and even ashamed of her medical illness. Instead of congratulating her for making a successful recovery from the operation, he berated her for coming to his office so late given the red flags during her worrisome ultrasound results three years ago, and taking so long to schedule the surgery after his strong suggestion. Not only was he unhappy with her delay, but he actually told her that "you had better listen to everything I say from now on if you want to get better." When she had jokingly mentioned how large her scar was, he aggressively implied that it was her own fault due to her reluctance to pursue the proper medical procedures that had been instructed to her.

My mother is a well-educated but traditional Chinese woman. Growing up, she had turned to Chinese herbs, remedies and other medicines in her times of illness. When she experienced bouts of menstrual pain, she took herbal soups to help ease her pain. She utilized herbal patches for her bumps and bruises. When she started ailing with back pains and sore tightness of her body from age and overwork, she scheduled herself for acupuncture and massage therapies. When her children became sick, she made herbal teas and Chinese medicinal soups to help alleviate the symptoms. She was never averse to Western medicine — she had always made frantic appointments for us and for herself when we showed any signs of serious illness — but the traditional, cultural remedies always brought her comfort and security. To her, Chinese medicine was as integral and natural as grabbing that bag of cough drops at the first signs of a sore throat and sniffles.

When they found abnormalities — nothing alarming, just something to check out — in a routine check-up three years ago, she had scampered away in avoidance when the words biopsy, needles and neck were put together due to her fear of pain. Eventually, after so much patient coaxing and remonstrating threats, I finally (gently, of course) twisted her arm to get that biopsy before I left for medical school. When her diagnosis confirmed both her physician's and my worries, she became hesitant about pursuing the next steps. Her continual disappointing experiences with the surgeons — one told her "you'll come back sooner or later" after she mentioned she wanted to wait, while another ridiculed her for her desire to pursue concurrent Chinese therapies — strongly dissuaded her from making any tangible plans.

Instead, she turned to what she knew well, to the prescriptions and medicinal remedies of Chinese medicine. She tried acupuncture and daily soups with sulfur. I was skeptical, but I opted to make a deal with her. If biopsies did not illustrate improvements after a few months, she had to pursue surgery. I huffed a huge sigh of relief when she finally found a surgeon who sat down and explained to her the significance of her disease, the reasons for such urgency for resection, and the steps that were involved.

And I was enraged for my mother. These physicians ignored my mother's concerns and failed to educate her about her own disease because they felt that not having surgery was completely out of the question. In their minds, there was no point explaining all the minutiae to her because she just did not get it, and it would not matter anyway. They already knew surgery provided her with the best outcome, so why wouldn't she do it? They had deemed Chinese medicine such a ludicrous alternative that it not only reflected her educational incompetence as a patient, but that there was absolutely no value in even discussing it.

It wasn't that my mother would not have agreed to the surgery sooner, but more that no one bothered to consider what she defined as a good clinical outcome and what constituted her quality of life. No one bothered to learn that she read online that she could develop long-term depression and lethargy after the operation, and she was terrified that she would be unable to be active and take care of her children. After all, being capable of supporting her family was absolutely necessary for her. No one bothered to find out that she had always been sensitive to medications, and she did not want to take hormones for the rest of her life. No one bothered to consider that being open to the matter of Chinese medicine would have made her much more comfortable with both the physician and the therapeutic options.

When did these things not become important? When did the clinical survival become so much more important that these "silly concerns?" When did our definition of a competent doctor outrank the different needs of our patients?

So what does it really mean to be a doctor? Do we decide what's best for our patients as medical experts? Do we yield to every patient's requests and needs in order to completely accommodate them? Or is there a way for us to meet at the middle? And if so, how do we achieve that through our training?

Questions

1. Do you believe it is important for clinicians to receive training in complementary and alternative medicine? How would you react to the author's mother in this narrative? Would you attempt to change her mind, or would you respect her autonomy? Is there a way to do both?

2. Have your opinions ever been disregarded by patients? How did this make you feel? Do you think patients feel the same way when their opinions are disregarded by clinicians?

3. This narrative reminds us why open communication is vital in the doctor-patient relationship. However, the author believes her mother desired not only open communication, but also open acceptance of the validity of her complementary remedies. Do you feel it is appropriate for clinicians to validate treatments that are outside of the ethos of their branch of medicine, especially if they are conflicting? Why or why not?

—Evan Torline

Breaking Down the Barrier

February 18, 2015

Pratik Kanabur
Virginia Tech Carilion School of Medicine
Class of 2018

I AM AN ENGINEERING graduate. My rigorous education has taught me that when presented with a problem, I should systematically narrow down solutions to figure out the best possible one.

During my second week of medical school I had my first standardized patient encounter. I felt very pleased with myself when I walked out the door after having asked the patient specific questions about her foot pain and been rewarded with the details of her worries. I figured that since she was complaining about her foot, I would fix the problem after I obtained the necessary skills. That's how it works right? It's how my engineering education had taught me to think.

But I could not have been more wrong. The professor quickly reprimanded me for not asking the question of *why*. Why was my patient worried about her foot pain? I personally thought that was none of my business; it isn't normal to ask personal questions, I believed. And so, at the time, I shrugged my shoulders and made note to prod a bit more next time.

During my next standardized patient encounter, I remembered to ask why. Why was my patient worried about her hip pain?

She told me she was concerned because her mother had needed hip surgery a few years ago. Okay, I thought, this time I nudged enough to obtain more information without getting too personal about her family. Wrong again. I was told I had still had not delved properly into my patient's emotional story. My professor told me to ask more why questions. Why did your mom go through hip surgery? How did she recover?

Dumbfounded, I asked, "What gives us this right to ask something so private?"

He simply responded: "The white coat."

As a physician, we are honored with the right — and the duty — to not only prod the patient for more information, but also to courageously break down the barriers that define social nicety. We were expected and judged on our ability to ask a series of intimate questions. To ask *why*.

During my first-year clinical experience, I was asked to obtain a patient's history. I asked her to tell me in her own words about her recent diabetes diagnosis. With a confused look, she asked me if I didn't want to know about her lab values or her medication immediately. She later told me she deeply appreciated my style of questioning, my willingness to listen and no-rush attitude. She talked about how she loved to eat.

Hmm, I thought, this was a good place to practice my prodding. As if the floodgates had opened, soon she was crying and telling me that she was feeling severely depressed because diabetes had taken away the last thing she loved. Luckily the doctor came into the room at that time, and she was able to talk to her and refer her to a psychiatrist.

It is always difficult to walk into a complete stranger's room and be comfortable enough to ask such personal questions. Often there are many differences in education, personality and culture that muddle relationships and make it hard to break barriers.

That day I realized how important it is to obtain as much information as possible from the patient and to form a connection with another human being. As a student doctor, I have to learn to gauge whether it is best to let patients break the barrier, open their floodgates, and swim through their feelings, or whether I should throw them a rope, ask them focused questions, and tug them back to the shore. When should I ask why? Regardless of the circumstances, always listen to the patient because they are the ones telling us the diagnosis. And never be afraid to ask just one more *why*.

Questions

1. The author had to put aside the systematic problem solving that he learned from his engineering background so that he could connect with his patient. What past training or habits do you foresee might interfere with how you think about your future patients and their concerns?

2. How can we ensure that our "prodding" has the best intentions — to maximize the quality of care for our patients — without simply appealing to our curiosity or nosiness?

3. What other privileges, aside from the privilege to ask our patients very personal questions, will our white coats afford us? Are there any privileges of which you may be hesitant to take advantage? How can we maintain respect for our patients as we break down these barriers?

—Tolulope Omojokun

A Case for Inclusive Language

April 1, 2015

Ria Pal
University of Rochester School of Medicine and Dentistry
Class of 2018

"AND DO YOU HAVE a husband at home?"
"A wife, actually."

"Oh, excuse me. And how long have you been with your mate?" the physician answered. He was unflustered and looked expectantly at the female standardized patient sitting across from him. For the remainder of the interview, when it came up again briefly, the physician referred to the patient's wife as her mate.

In just the last few months, I've read a thoughtful essay contrasting biological sex and gender and a piece on the shortcomings of health care providers in caring for queer patients.[1] Literature on discrimination (particularly sexism, racism and heterosexism) in medical school and in the medical field is easy to find.[2,3,4] Now a growing body of academic work, anecdotes and political history has revealed that medical education is comfortably rooted in a system that presumes traditionally privileged demographics: cis-gendered, heterosexual, slim, able, neurotypical, literate, white, male, wealthy. Often, what is not labeled as default is labeled as abnormal at best, and pathological at worst.

My chief concern is not in why we prioritize social justice — for my purposes, the equitable distribution of wealth, opportunity and privilege within a society — but rather, what steps can be taken to further it, particularly as students, novices to medicine's intensely hierarchical culture. Here, I'd like to examine the way that we use language: to include or to alienate, intentionally or from habit.

So what was problematic about the encounter above? A dictionary will tell you that "mate" and "spouse" are virtually synonymous, as are "lover" and "significant other." The standardized patient didn't get visibly upset. Most of us know, however, that these words carry distinct connotations, and that it takes a degree of self-assuredness to correct assumptions (perhaps more so the assumptions of someone in a position of relative power, like a health care provider). While many would view the encounter above as benign, that in itself points to the widespread acceptance of microaggression and the idea that it is the responsibility of the marginalized to educate. The patient may have answered, "No, I don't have a husband," and stopped there for fear of homophobia; the physician may have failed to collect pertinent information as a result of heteronormative language.

Moreover, the failure to outright recognize the patient's marriage, particularly in light of same-sex couples' fraught history and present, is callous. Denial of marriage as a civil right is one of many heavy oppressions that LGBT patients as a demographic are forced to bear, and which may play a role in their higher risks for several STIs, homelessness and suicide.

I'm convinced that to make progress toward alleviating health inequities, we need to actively change our language — at the bedside, in the lecture hall, in our homes. Political correctness is not the point. Critically thinking about language goes beyond doing the minimum and avoiding offense, and rather indicates genuine concern for those targeted. To be aware of language is to be aware of a fundamental measure of the status quo. Our choices of language are often unintentional, but almost always acknowledge deep-set assumptions. When someone uses sexual orientation and gender identification interchangeably in a speech or on a form, they may reveal biases or gaps in knowledge. In the words of a classmate, careless language is analogous to symptoms of disease. Careless language is a product of a larger scheme of how we differentially value others (whether it be racism or heterosexism), just as symptoms are produced by underlying pathology. Examining symptoms helps us to understand these larger problems. And within this analogy, a symptom, whether it is a high fever or the disappointment that follows hearing a slur, is itself the lived experience of the larger problem — it is the sting of feeling unwelcome, the nausea of degradation.

Think critically about language: the language that you use as well as the language that surrounds you. Is it inclusive? Is it informed?

Inclusive language is informed, stripped of assumptions, and intentionally represents diversity. An informed speaker has taken the time to learn preferred pronouns and allows the subject to self-identify. An unassuming speaker recognizes that family structures are diverse and that patients and peers come from wide varieties of cultures, financial means and educational levels, all of which impact communication and understanding. An intentional speaker incorporates all genders rather than addressing their audience with a bluntly divisive "ladies and gentlemen."

Learning to be more inclusive with one's own language is a constant process. Gracefully correcting oneself and accepting corrections is key to growth. So too is a persistent humility and openness; everyone should have the freedom to self-identify, without fear of judgment or stereotyping. It's only a beginning step, but adapting our language to be more inclusive is essential to being compassionate, competent physicians. While it might be slow going, I'm optimistic that it is achievable.

Questions

1. Think of an instance where you have made an assumption (either aloud or to yourself) about a patient's lifestyle, sexual orientation or gender. If you could go back and change that interaction, what would you do differently?

2. Until 1973, homosexuality was classified as a mental disorder. How do you think this historical heterosexism plays into encounters today between physicians and patients who identify as LGBT?

3. Does a health care provider need to know the sexual or gender orientation of a patient when that information won't directly impact care, such as a posttransition transgender female who is to undergo a cholecystectomy? Why or why not?

—Chelcie Soroka

Remembering What It Is Like Not to Know

April 26, 2015

Katie Taylor
Icahn School of Medicine at Mount Sinai
Class of 2016

A FEW WEEKS AGO, I was describing my team's discharge plan to the patient I had been following all week. We had found an anterior mediastinal mass on imaging, and the pulmonologist wanted to follow-up in a week after immunohistological staining came back. I told him we felt he was now stable, and that we would like him to follow up with the lung doctor as an outpatient within the week.

He asked me if he should return to the ER to get his appointment.

Noooo, I told him, the ER was the last place I wanted him to revisit. It was two days prior, utterly short of breath and with a lung full of fluid that he had barely walked into the ER before he was admitted to our medicine service. He said he didn't want to go there again either. We verbally orbited each other until finally he asked, "What is outpatient?"

A few weeks later, while on holiday break, my aunt asked me what a resident was, and did they have their MD? My parents asked, what *is* internal medicine, and isn't all medicine largely internal anyway?

I am two and a half years into this training, and yet already am disremembering what it is like to not have had this schooling, to be a non-medical student. I hear the talk, read the talk, try to write the talk, and then, suddenly, I am walking the talk. To my patients' and my own confusion. It must be what it is like to join the Marines, or live in a highly religious sect — they strip down all you know, and they build their new flock back up, using the same learned code and rituals, rights and responsibilities. Instead of "citizens" or "gentiles" or "Muggles," we call the non-initiated "patients."

I was consistently annoyed as a first-year medical student when lecturers used comically and needlessly medical terms — did they categorically need to use the word "tachycardic" instead of fast heart rate? It was, in fact, adding a syllable, and significantly worsening our comprehension. Lecturer after lecturer would liberally use jargon and then the all-confusing acronym, not knowing we were far closer to a layman than a professional. In one breath a pulmonologist spoke of RV, FEV1, FVC, the cardiologist of LVEFs, LAs and PMIs.

It was only a few months into my medical school career that I started donating biannually during Wikipedia's funding drive — I couldn't have survived these classes without Wikipedia-ing every third word on the slide.

And yet now, two and a half years later, my vocabulary has metamorphosed to a stunning degree. I catch myself saying "hypertension" instead of "high blood pressure." I hear myself speaking sentences littered with medical jargon in front of patients — my medical thoughts now flow most naturally in their medical linguistic domain, it seems — and I have to backtrack my way to the realm of common language and straightforward words.

It scares me how these two years have transmuted my speech and I only assume my thinking, too.

A part of me is excited by how much I have absorbed. Medicine has created a specific language to describe ailments, medications and symptomatology. It is important to accurately define and label a patient's consciousness as lethargic, obtunded or somnolent. Radiologists must precisely articulate the location of their findings. Clarity and specificity are vital.

And yet, it's been shown medical students become worse communicators through their years in medical school and are less able to understand patients' overall views on their health. In reviewing thousands of live and taped doctor-patient sessions, physicians consistently use medical terms patients don't understand and patients do not clarify either, due to intimidation and fear of looking uneducated. Up to half of patients leave a doctor's office unsure of what information was exchanged and what actions they were instructed to take to better their health.

The studies go on, and get more depressing: docs are distinctly poor listeners and explainers, patient interviewing has become embarrassingly abbreviated, and now less than five percent of a visit is used to even transmit information from doctor to patient. It's an overwhelming and grim topic that speaks forcefully to the skeleton of what the "art of doctoring" has become, and more broadly to what is rewarded throughout premedical and medical training and to the devaluation of talk, which occurs mostly in primary care physician offices.

For all this training affords me, I worry about what it takes away. I hope I can hold on to how unsettling and uncertain it is to be unwell and not to know the details of the diagnosis, if there is even a clear diagnosis to be made at all. That I may remember that things that seem so clear and self-evident to me may be obscure and peculiar to others. That the words I now know are my own narrow area of soon-to-be proficiency, and I couldn't follow a lawyer discussing a bank merger, or a plumber discussing pipes, any more than they could read a CT scan.

Or in other words, as I become a doctor, I hope I become equal parts translator and educator. For what good is this information stored inside me if no one knows that I am talking about.

Questions

1. Have you found yourself using medical jargon with friends and family who did not understand your terminology? How might their reactions in such situations differ from our patients' reactions when they are similarly bewildered?

2. What advantages and disadvantages are there to having a separate vocabulary to describe our patients' conditions? Is jargon really necessary in medical culture?

3. How can we talk with our patients in a way that ensures they understand us without becoming condescending toward them?

—Tolulope Omojokun

Burnout

How Medical School Taught Me to Put Studying Second

February 4, 2014

Samuel Scott
University of Toledo College of Medicine
Class of 2015

YOU KNOW YOU HAVE a problem when you can't fall asleep at night. That's where I was nearing at the end of anatomy in my first year of medical school. I couldn't sleep because I was terrified of what the next day held. My sympathetic nervous system was on full alert, ready to handle the next day. The only thing between the next day and me was a night of sleep that seemed harder and harder to get.

In "The Chronicles of Narnia," C.S. Lewis remarks that sleep is something that becomes more difficult the harder you try to accomplish it. This was the curse of my predicament. I was exhausted and in dire need of rest at the end of each day, but held captive by what "could" happen the next day.

In a follow-up visit with my pediatrician over winter break, I had some testing done that revealed some unanticipated results. Though I had been diagnosed with ADHD in grade school, my pattern of inattention and easy distractibility was more consistent with an anxiety disorder than ADHD. With further questioning and history taking, it became obvious that I was a classic case of generalized anxiety disorder.

It wasn't something that was created from the rigors of medical school; it was something *revealed* for what it was by the rigors of medical school. I had been able to get by to this point on sheer intelligence and good test taking skills, but now I was at the point of not being able to function.

I started some medication, but I fumbled my way through the end of the year. Things didn't get much better. It wasn't until the second year of medical school that I realized that my health had to come first in life.

Immunity and Infection is the second hardest class I've ever taken in my life. I've never worked so hard at anything, let alone work that hard just to fail repeatedly. I didn't feel as utterly incompetent as physical chemistry made me feel, but I felt just as helpless. Fifteen hours of class and active-brain-based studying a day and I couldn't get closer to passing than half a point.

Eleven weeks into a 13-week course and I couldn't get over that hump. I did all the hard work, ignored my mental health and sucked it up and that got me to within half a point of passing week after week. I finally quit. Those last two weeks of class I essentially quit studying. I slept until I woke up in the morning. I spent an average of two hours reading my bible and praying. I casually flipped through notes during the day but compared to my previous efforts, I might as well have not been studying.

What happened might have been Divine intervention, a stroke of luck or simply a consequence of taking care of my own head. I saw my grade jump 15 percentage points in those last two weeks.

After that brutal gauntlet and quitting before I reached the finish line, the most important thing I learned during that class wasn't which antibiotic to use, but rather that I had to take care of myself before studying. That meant good sleep hygiene, eating healthy, regular exercise, spiritual health and some medications.

After making some adjustments I saw major improvements in my quality of life, which was important because some unexpected life events that were out of my control were just around the bend leading up to Step 1. Without those changes and the help of my friends and administrators, I wouldn't have finished the year.

Some medical students keep studying as their number one priority in life, but for me it was a matter of passing and failing. I had to take care of my mental health first.

Questions

1. In what ways can you care for yourself and your own mental health during your medical education?

2. Are you open with your fellow classmates about the difficulties of medical school? How can we as students change and improve medical education to promote student wellness?

3. Do you feel your medical school supports the need for self-care for its medical students? Would you feel comfortable telling people you needed to dial back a bit in order to take care of your mental health?

—Aleena Paul

Do They Teach Fear in Medical School?

April 4, 2014

Ajay Koti
University of South Florida Morsani College of Medicine
Class of 2017

R *OOM ONE*

Wendy Smith had thinning hair, penciled-in eyebrows, and a frame so thin that you could see, in painstaking detail, bluish-grey veins emanating from beneath her pale skin. Cancer had taken so much from her that she almost didn't look human.

But the feeling in the room was extremely human. Fear — palpable fear. Fear made all the more palpable because this was an aggressive, rare form of cancer. Fear made all the more palpable because she was young, only in her early 30s. Fear made all the more palpable because the cancer had been discovered during postnatal care following the birth of her first child.

Motherhood ... and chemotherapy.

It was hard not to detect a little desperation in her husband's voice as he kept asking about new, experimental treatments he had read about in his own research. It was chilling to think that the notion of single fatherhood had undoubtedly crossed his mind.

Room Two

Susan James was older and had already experienced breast cancer, which had recurred for the umpteenth time after numerous rounds of treatment. However, the tumor in her breast was not the reason for today's visit.

Today's visit was to tell her about the tumor in her bladder.

Her visage was blank, almost hollow. The word "surgery" snapped her out of her shock. Waving her hands with tears welling in her eyes, she said she didn't want to hear about surgery; she didn't even want to think about it. She had already been under the knife half a dozen times, she had endured

247

radiation and chemotherapy, and now she had to consider surgery to remove her bladder — it was just too much. Too much, at least for today. The doctor wisely pulled back, consoled Susan, and urged her to go home, to be with her family for the holidays, and maybe even to take a vacation. Decide in the New Year. No rush.

Room Three

John Peters was different. A veteran of cancer fights with the scars to prove it, John was nonchalant about his medical condition, nodding along to some of the doctor's medical jargon and tossing out some of his own, a demonstration of the expertise he had accumulated in the course of his treatments. As we left the exam room, he casually asked for a syringe with some saline solution so that he could flush out his own nephrostomy tube, which, he noted in a matter-of-fact way, had become clogged after bleeding from his kidney.

Soapbox

It's hard to imagine a more appropriate setting for patient-centered care than an oncology clinic. The doctor I shadowed employed many of its humanistic tenets to these three patients: sitting by their side, giving them a gentle touch on the shoulder, and conveying a strong sense of optimism without once veering into the dangerous, and often heartbreaking, territory of false hope. These qualities of good bedside manner are smart tactics, but they are even more effective in the context of a larger strategy that places the patient's values, priorities, and dignity at the forefront.

Still, there is a tendency, on the part of some, to dismiss patient-centered care: being "extra nice" to patients is a quaint concept, but ultimately irrelevant and even naïve. With the pressures of the health care system, it is often thought to be entirely more efficient and important for doctors to focus on getting patients cured and out the door. *We didn't come to medical school to hold people's hands — we came to treat them.* I've sensed this attitude not only from practicing physicians, but also, on occasion, from fellow students. Intellectually, I know I should respect this view, just as I expect my more humanistic motivations to be given credence.

In reality, I have a hard time with this.

How can you treat people if you don't understand them?

How can you treat people if you don't even care to understand them?

Perhaps it comes down to how each of us defines success in medicine. Money in the bank? Social status? I am fond of joking that my bleeding-heart liberal Messiah complex will lead me to a career as a psychiatrist in a North Dakota prison, but I have few illusions in reality. I won't pretend that I will eschew the rich socioeconomic perks that come with a medical career.

However, my main goal is different. I want to be meaningful and useful to my patients. I want to be a person they trust — a bedrock of support they can count on in the moments of confusion and uncertainty — in the moments of fear. I want my patients to feel like they're going to be all right before I pull out a prescription pad. The patients I met in the oncology clinic were only there for office visits — their tumors didn't shrink by the end of their appointments, but there was a sense of peace in their faces that wasn't there twenty minutes earlier. Their cancer didn't get any better, but, their fear did.

I don't know — maybe I'm being naïve.

I'll take my chances.

Questions

1. Think of a time that you have sensed a patient's fear. How did you react to the patient, and what did you do or say? Did the patient's fear affect your ability to provide empathetic care? Why or why not?

2. Now, think of a time that you were afraid during medical school. Were you afraid of something happening to you, or something happening to someone else? How did you cope with these feelings? What would you want someone to say to you if you were afraid?

3. What do you think the author means by "teaching fear"? Is there a role of medical schools in teaching students how to cope with fear? What are some ways that a medical school can teach these skills?

4. Do you think repeated confrontations with fear, as the author illustrates in these three clinical vignettes, can have a long-term effect on the well-being of physicians-in-training? Do you think fear is a component of burnout? Why or why not?

—Sasha Yakhkind

Idea Worship:
Mindfulness in Medical School

May 22, 2014

Andrew Kadlec
Medical College of Wisconsin
Class of 2017

*E*YES CLOSED, *shallow breaths.*
A serene, deserted beach in the south of France, in the near future. Children playing far away in a field, their laughter carried by the wind to nearby cliffs, where it glances off the soaring cliffs and echoes softly in my ears. Waves gently sweeping across the land, creating transient, unique impressions in the sand ... again and again. My fingers slowly intertwine with those of another, and I am gratified by a warmth that envelops me. I grasp more tightly, dig my toes into the wet sand, and gaze out at the horizon.

As I write these lines, I admit that I feel the allure of this romanticized sketch, even though my purpose is to now caution against such Elysian abstraction. A propensity to fantasize is built into human nature; it is the reason we escape into virtual realities through books, movies, video games and even our careers. And while envisioning that beach in France certainly enchants the senses, what is the effect of absorbing oneself into such idealized images?

As a part of "The Healer's Art," an elective course for first-year medical students, we were given the opportunity to practice "mindfulness," by silencing our thoughts and turning our minds to the present. It was neither simple nor simplistic, and I began to wonder why we have difficulty tuning out future-oriented thoughts about our ambitions, our fears, even what we want to eat tonight — anything but the present scene. This inability to fully devote our minds and ourselves to the present is particularly germane to medical training. Given the amount of time that must be invested in both education and training — years that often seem to stretch indefinitely ahead of us — the medical path naturally encourages its travelers to engage in constant projection into the future, to worship the idea of arriving at some distant goal, be it geographical, financial or professional.

As medical students, it will often be tempting to imagine ourselves in a future time and place regarding our careers, as well as our lives, in general. Physicians who are a little farther down the road than we are state that this kind of idea worship will accompany us throughout our professional career, either when considering ourselves ("Should I take that job? Will it allow me to get to the 'next level?'") or our patients ("What will his clinical outcome look like?"). This projection can motivate us to work hard now to become the doctor we envision in our mind's eye. After all, we need to plan and position ourselves for success, and it is essential to the well-being of our patients that we think about where we would like to be in 10 to 20 years. In doing so, we come to appreciate what particular skills or interests we possess that will best suit us for a certain field and enable us to best serve our patients.

Despite the benefits of visualizing future scenarios, such projection can also inhibit one's ability to focus on the present, as well as increase personal anxiety. I sometimes find myself not listening to a patient as much as I should be, instead contemplating, "Could I see myself doing the surgery that would help this lady? Maybe I should set up an opportunity to find out about that." By not listening to this patient, I rob both of us the opportunity to establish personal contact and, for me, to learn as much as possible about the case in order to best handle a similar one in the future. If I do not pay attention to the present, I am not best preparing myself to be a compassionate and competent physician. Constantly thinking about the future does not necessarily translate into being more successful in the future.

A subtle trap occurs when we do find ourselves dwelling on future possibilities. Danielle Ofri, MD, PhD, who delivered a compelling talk at our school a few months ago, described this cognitive nearsightedness — she said that what we imagine initially as the diagnosis, and around which we establish a treatment plan, is given such preference that our vision is reduced. As a result, we may miss other likely, potentially more threatening possibilities. We need to be wary of this trap and continually bring ourselves back to the present, focusing on a new piece of history or a new symptom that could lend weight to a different diagnosis.

Orienting our outlook and actions around our initial thought is not simply relevant to patient care; it also has the potential to impact our own lives. In "Mere Christianity," C.S. Lewis states that, "The thrill you feel on first seeing some delightful place dies away when you really go to live there..." There is always a discord between what we imagine something will be like and what it actually is like. I spent weeks during the first semester of medical school envisioning the exact specialty that would be the best fit for me. As I have discovered more about otolaryngology, my view of it has changed significantly. Fortunately, it has piqued my interest even more, but so have other specialities, and much of the anxiety that I felt during those weeks could have been lessened if I had not given so much weight to a single idea. I have been told that this conflict between our present ideas and the future reality will always exist. Take, for example, the shift in urological interventions, as described by my brother — many surgeons are not doing procedures now for which they trained in residency, and many are also doing procedures now that they never did in residency. We need to realize that what we imagine life will be like is just that — an exploration of hypothetical possibilities, not a single absolute certainty — and that we must always be aware of and receptive to other options.

Isn't medical school at least slightly different than you had imagined, in terms of the people, the institution and the courses? And wait, wasn't getting into medical school what we envisioned as "making it," allowing us to finally do what we wanted to do? Another major issue with this type of anticipatory thinking is our propensity to constantly modify the idea, each new fantasy giving rise to and slipping into the next. We imagine one scenario, and then find ourselves within it, only to move on to the next new scenario — the one in which we imagine we will be truly happy.

Becoming a full-fledged physician takes a long time, and our careers will hopefully continue long past the point of initial autonomy. Habitually thinking about the future only makes the path seem longer and interferes with our ability to appreciate the present. As medical students, it's critical that we take time to enjoy the steps along the way and the awesome privilege to learn about the fascinatingly complex human body. Do what you can to focus on the present, whether it is asking a patient deeper questions about his or her medical history or hobbies, writing down something new that you learned today, or simply exercising (there is nothing like a sore body to turn your mind to the present).

Maybe I will discover one day that the beach in France does not look the same as it did in my mental travel guide. Surely I cannot determine today whether the idea-turned-reality will be better, or worse, or simply different. I will have to wait to find out. For now, I will try to turn my gaze from the horizon to the beach, because the person I love, sitting next to me right now, the patient in the waiting room, the here and now in all of its capacious, rich glory, deserve just as much of my study and contemplation.

Questions

1. What strategies do you use or have you seen used to reconnect to the present and stay mindful? Do you feel that those strategies allow you and your colleagues to better care for patients?

2. Can you think of a time that a patient helped you to appreciate the current moment?

3. Are there any opportunities in your medical school to explore mindfulness? Why have you chosen or not chosen to explore these self-care techniques?

—Natalie Wilcox

How to Find the Strength to Keep Going: Words of Advice from a Third-Year

July 24, 2014

Jarna Shah
University of Illinois at Chicago College of Medicine
Class of 2015

IT'S 4 A.M., AND I'm sitting in the student call room eating dinner during a particularly busy night. A burrito has never tasted this good.

Here's the truth: medical school isn't glamorous. More often than not, it involves long hours and late nights. There will be days where you come home and fall asleep before eating dinner. There will be 10-hour surgical cases with no bathroom breaks and mornings where rounds take five hours. You will spend hours on hold with social services and you will run around the hospital like the gawky medical student you are, trying to track down paperwork.

On the roughest days and latest of nights, it is hard to find the strength to crawl into bed, wake up in the morning, and go back to the hospital. Tough experiences and unfriendly coworkers can aggravate that inner self-loathing and make you feel disgusted at yourself. A lack of rest, a newly developed caffeine habit, and an unhealthy dependence on granola bars doesn't help.

So, what do you do to keep going?

I write down my memories and keep them in a jar to remind me why I am here. It serves as a break from my frantic struggles of transitioning between rotations and trying to choose a career and plan for the upcoming year.

This may seem a bit childish. A bit too nostalgic and perhaps a tad immature, but I can't tell you how many times I have needed these little things this year.

I can't forget how my very first patient on the wards told me that I was going to be a good doctor. I grin when I think of my little pediatric patient learning my name and telling me good morning every day when I went to see him. We watched Harry Potter together. And I won't soon forget the words of a terminal cancer patient as he told me that my eyes sparkled like somebody in love. In a way, he was right. I was in love with what I did every day.

On my wall, I have a paper EKG strip with the exact moment when my patient with an irregular atrial fibrillation jumped back into a normal rhythm. It reminds me that human physiology is kind of amazing.

I connected with a patient over the socks I was wearing. A resident told me (jokingly) that she would fail me on my evaluation, just so I would have to repeat the rotation and spend more time with her. In my broken Spanish, I had the privilege of helping a woman give birth to a beautiful healthy baby. I've even accidentally met my little sister's math teacher in the pediatric clinic during spring break.

I won't forget the urologist salsa dancing with the scrub nurse in the OR before the beginning of a long case. I told a scared little girl stories about orthopedic surgeons and their space suits, right before she fell asleep on the operating table. I've had a resident physically boot me out of the hospital on a slow call night because "it's Friday night, and you're young, and you should go have a good time."

Not all of my cherished memories are cheerful. I remember my last interactions with a patient before she passed away during the night. I wish I would have gone back to her room that night before leaving. Consoling a resident as she tearfully told me about a toddler who was dying of meningococcemia; listening to frustrated parents snipe at me and threaten to leave the hospital against medical advice; being chased down the hall by a psychotic patient in her wheelchair, swearing angrily — I remember sometimes feeling so unbelievably useless.

There is nothing glorious about rushing to your first code blue. There is little beauty in watching a patient's dying rattling breaths. There are no words to express the pain of watching the delivery of a brain-dead full-term infant. After events like these, there is only a gaping hole of disillusionment and discontent that wraps around you like a suffocating blanket.

I save my stories to remind me to feel in a time when I become so numb. For when I become immune to daily complaints of back pain and intermittent headaches. For when I forget the narratives that bring my patients to life, and I forget what brought me here.

I have been given the privilege to be privy to the tales of so many individuals. It is a gift that I can't afford to squander. There is no parallel to the amount of trust a patient puts in my hands even though I am not yet a physician. With each passing day, I fall more in love with my job and my career. I hope those of you in medicine or planning to pursue a career in medicine feel the same way.

I urge you all to keep a jar, whether it is a physical container, a metaphorical room in your mind, or even notes or photos on your phone. Keep a jar with your most precious thoughts and anecdotes — they don't have to be related to medicine. Fill it with the joy and the fear and the anticipation that each day brings. Stay upbeat and optimistic even when the real world begs to differ. Don't forget why you are where you are. Don't become immune to the pain and joy and suffering that surrounds you in each hospital setting. Remember. Feel. And keep going.

Questions

1. What do you do to navigate the stressful and sometimes numbing experiences we encounter as medical students? Is it enough? Explain.

2. What is your best memory from the wards? What is your worst memory? How have those experiences affected you personally and professionally?

3. In recent years, more research has been published on physician and physician-in-training burnout. Do you think this is an inevitably natural outcome as a result of the hours, experiences, and professional stress that is placed on health care professionals, or that it is something that can be avoided? Explain.

4. What do you think is the right balance between emotional connection and emotional detachment toward patients? Are you more worried about feeling too much, or feeling too little toward patients? How do you plan to keep an open-hearted attitude toward patients?

—Vikas Bhatt

Wounded Healers

November 14, 2014

Ajay Koti
University of South Florida Morsani College of Medicine
Class of 2017

K AITLYN ELKINS WAS A medical student at the Wake Forest School of Medicine in North Carolina and a member of the Class of 2015. She excelled academically, was named the valedictorian of her high school class and graduated summa cum laude from Campbell University. She wrote poetry in her free time. She had a cat, lovingly named Gatito. On April 11, 2013, just weeks before beginning her clinical rotations, Kaitlyn Elkins took her own life. She left behind a note revealing her battle with depression, a struggle that was hidden from her family for years.

A few months ago, in separate incidents, two medical school graduates in the early weeks of internship jumped to their deaths. An estimated 300 to 400 physicians die annually from suicide, and as many as 21.2% of medical students suffer from depression.[1,2]

At first glance, the genesis of this problem seems obvious: stress. Beginning with the application process and increasing with cutthroat tests and hours of toiling away in the wards, medical school can be a crucible of intensity. Students are under more pressure than ever to achieve, particularly because residencies haven't kept pace with growing medical schools. Things don't look too stable on the other side of graduation either: tectonic shifts in insurance markets, new payment and delivery systems, reductions in reimbursement, student loan debt, and tens of millions of patients added to already bursting patient panels. This is an intimidating list of challenges, and it is telling that an article labeling ours as "the most miserable profession" went viral in medical circles.[3] A kind of malaise has settled over the field.

The "stress" argument is convenient. It's logical and neat, and its conclusion is fairly obvious — namely, that we need to reduce medical student and physician stress. Who wouldn't get behind that?

Convenient though it may be, a review of the literature and a little soul-searching reveal this argument to be incomplete at best. Plenty of occupations are stressful, and while we all experience stress, most students are not depressed and will not commit suicide.[4] Personal distress (i.e. depression) has been shown to be distinct from burnout in medical students.[5] One article also found that depressed medical students are more likely to have had a pre-medical school episode of depression than non-depressed students and that medicine seemed to "unwitting[ly] select ... predisposed students."[6]

Depression among medical professionals is perhaps more deeply rooted than we'd care to admit. A landmark study of physician attributes uncovered a whole range of psychological vulnerabilities: self-criticism, a refusal to seek help, pessimism, passivity, self-doubt and feelings of inferiority, among others.[7] The authors suggested that these intrinsic characteristics were more predictive of personal and psychological dysfunction later in life. Stressors, personal or professional, may only be triggers that expose deeper wounds.

Wounded healers. It's a concept from Jungian psychology thought to be inspired by the story of Chiron, a centaur in Greek mythology who was renowned for his skills as a healer. Chiron was wounded by a poisoned arrow but his immortal status sustained him despite the incurable wound. He was thus condemned to spend eternity roaming the earth in agonizing pain, healing everybody but himself. Jung applied the concept mostly to psychoanalysts, but the phenomena of depression and suicide among medical students and doctors suggest that we too fit into this archetype.

These wounds present a double-edged sword. On one hand, they can be powerful motivators. Johnson suggested that some physicians pursue their craft in response to negative childhood experiences, whether from illness, trauma or neglect.[8] Vulnerability may also allow for more empathetic and meaningful patient interactions. Dr. Alice Flaherty, author of "The Midnight Disease," has repeatedly stated that her experiences with bipolar disorder have made her a better caregiver.[9] It has also been demonstrated that physicians with a history of depression are significantly more likely to investigate suicidal ideation in depressed patients than physicians without a history of depression.[10] Healers are better equipped to care for the sick if they have experienced sickness firsthand.

But the same qualities that lead to success in medicine can have tragic consequences, as evidenced by the alarming statistics on depression and suicide in the profession. This leads to a complicated question: what can we do about it? Few medical students with depression actually seek out treatment; when asked for reasons, they cite lack of time (48 percent), lack of confidentiality (37 percent), stigma (30 percent), cost (28 percent) and fear of documentation on their academic records (24 percent).[11]

Fortunately, medical schools nationwide have been making efforts to address this crisis. Academically, the shift to now ubiquitous pass/fail grading systems was partially motivated by a desire to reduce levels of student stress, anxiety and depression. Other resources at the student level like mindfulness training, peer mentoring, service opportunities and student wellness groups are all welcome developments. Further, the Liaison Committee on Medical Education now mandates the provision of counseling services delivered by professionals who are kept separate from students' academic experience. Some schools go a step further and provide financial assistance if and when mental health care is indicated. Though counseling services are guaranteed, the jury is still out on their efficacy, underscoring the need for research in this area. And, given the aforementioned self-identified barriers to treatment, medical students would benefit from greater assurance that the use of mental health services is confidential and completely separate from academic records.

But the most meaningful change is not institutional. It's cultural. Even in medical circles, depression remains poorly understood and stigma is rampant. Fifty-six percent of depressed students suspect they would lose the respect of their colleagues if their depression became public; 83 percent of depressed students suspect that faculty would view them as unfit for their responsibilities.[12] One student confided to me that he had stopped attending a depression support group because it was held in a building on campus, and that he didn't want to risk being recognized by any students or faculty. Changing the culture of medicine to be more supportive and accepting is a slow process, but it is also the part that we can most directly influence. It's also necessary — how can we hope to care for patients if we don't take care of our own?

Kaitlyn Elkins' mother, Rhonda, was devastated by the loss of her daughter. She wrote a book, "My Bright Shining Star," and started a blog.[13,14] The website is a chronicle of her grief, expressing emotions that range from shock and anger to misty-eyed remembrance. Reading it is a gut-wrenching experience. Rhonda also became a tireless advocate for mental health awareness, bravely sharing her experiences with others. She even posted on the online forums at the Student Doctor Network, offering support to medical students. She touched the lives of countless people, many of whom she would never even meet.

On August 29, 2014, Rhonda Elkins took her own life. She was 54 years old.

Author's note: My thanks to the Elkins family for sharing Kaitlyn and Rhonda with us and for allowing me to tell some of their stories here.

Questions

1. Would you agree with the statement that many medical students and health professionals are "wounded healers"?

2. What would you do if a colleague showed signs of depression or expressed suicidal thoughts?

3. Is vulnerability a component of mental health, or part of the human condition? How might this change how we approach the mental health of physicians-in-training?

4. Does open awareness of mental health allow us to have better interactions with our patients? With our peers?

5. What qualities or processes should medical education adopt to make room for personal vulnerabilities?

—Nisha Pradhan

Rite of Passage

February 1, 2015

Nita Chen
Albany Medical College
Class of 2017

T HE SNOW HAS FULLY started in Albany. With coldness sprinkling its physical manifestations in flurries, the imminence of winter and another year's end are tangible. The shuffling students that occupy the classrooms thin as more and more of us choose to study within the warmths of our homes and snuggies. The second year of medical school has truly been a test of endurance and resilience. The two-week themes and examinations have certainly been another challenge to adjust to, many of us exploring and adapting different study strategies in attempts to maximize our time for the ominous Step 1 studying.

Meanwhile, I hear the echoes of the now third-year students as my fellow peers divulge their knowledge to the eager and nervous first-years that plead for advice. It is almost if I were listening to a playback of my first-year anxieties. Having almost blown through first semester at a lightning pace, it is natural to talk about the metamorphosis that we have all undergone. Looking back, the plasticity inherent in all of us has allowed for extraordinary adjustment to the increasingly hefty academic demand that has been lumped onto our mental plates within these short few months. It feels strange and even dissociative to me at times that the obstacles that we encountered just 365 days ago now seem so ... trivial.

As I hear and watch my now seasoned second-year classmates interact with these doe-eyed underclassmen, I feel a sense of worry and sometimes even slight frustration at the attitudes that are occasionally expressed.

You have so much time, you don't even know.

Don't worry. Don't stress so much. Second year is so much harder.

We had to go through it, too, so it's not like it's impossible. Just hang on, and you'll get the hang of things soon.

I recall a sort of deja vu to the words delivered to us by our now third-years, and I remember that frustration I felt regarding those similar comments. I remember the sense of isolation and helplessness at their attempt to put our difficulties in perspective. Yes, I know each year becomes progressively difficult in a different way. In the long run, the examinations and grades acquired during our pre-clinical years are simply another pebble in the mountain of obstacles we must climb, but in that moment, being told this didn't relieve any of my stress. In fact, it made it worse. I felt overwhelmed and confused by the chafing changes of medical school, and the knowledge that it will only get worse didn't exactly ease my nail-biting worries. It's not that the upperclassmen weren't helpful. They have been very reliable shoulders that we leaned on, providing their thoughtful ears to our complaints and venting. But along those lines, I also sensed a sort of necessity being upheld to the difficulties that we experience — a rite of passage, of sorts.

And it makes sense. Without rigorous training, the bastion of medical excellence would surely crumple like forgotten days-old pastries. But let's be honest, casting aside the financial burdens that some of us have placed upon ourselves, climbing out of medical school relatively unscathed and somewhat whole is already tough enough as it is. Surviving the curriculum, keeping abreast with the ever-changing new medications whilst remembering all their seemingly nonsensical names, balancing life outside of medicine — are these not enough as rites of passage? Is it really necessary for students to have to prove to each other that we are intelligent, capable individuals? At the end of this long four-year journey, we all stand shoulder to shoulder as equals, as doctors.

As human beings, we seek validation of our abilities and respect from others. With that, it is only natural that we find it fair that our following underclassmen undergo the same rigors and hardships that we endured as we did, just as our predecessors often expect of us. In some sort of distorted logic, the suffering and struggle that we had to writhe through in order to get where we are has become integrated as one of the numerous requirements for us to confirm our skills and validate the efforts in our endeavors. I am sure we have all heard the core of the phrase, *you haven't experienced first year until you get to x theme or met y professor.* On some level, medical school will always entail shared obstacles that we all must learn to take in stride. However, there are so many ways that we can help each other make these experiences less painful without impeding growth.

I think there are so many things that the medical educational system needs to change in order to not only improve medical care, but also to mold more wholesome medical professionals. This change can start with us, the medical students. We must change our belief that being overwhelmed and frustrated is a necessary aspect of medical school. Let's start with being kind to ourselves and to each other. Let's can start by believing that success doesn't have to come with martyrdom and suffering. Let's start by allowing our peers to lean on each other.

Questions

1. How can medical students cope with the inherent stresses of medical school while still maintaining a passion for learning and patient care?

2. What are the pros and cons to the "overwhelming" and "frustrating" aspects of medical school training? Are these aspects important to becoming a physician, or are they detrimental?

3. How can upperclass students better support preclinical students in enduring this "rite of passage" in medical school?

4. How can we best distinguish the benefits of tradition and the limits of historicity as pertains to our own "rite of passage" in medical school and beyond?

—Steven Lange

Booster

March 19, 2015

Jennifer Tsai
Warren Alpert Medical School of Brown University
Class of 2018

F OR ME, HEPATITIS B booster shots feel pretty much as pleasant as being sucker punched in the arm. You can imagine that it didn't inspire much elation when I scrolled through my calendar to see, spelled out in big red letters, a reminder for "Hep B #3."

Now, as I reflect, this reminder feels like a victory of sorts.

When you are told during medical school orientation that you must be re-immunized for hepatitis B, you are sent to undergo a three-dose course: zero months, one month, six months. I remember making those appointments while standing next to a shaded window, looking out into the brutish heat of an August in Providence. I remember thinking that six months felt so far away. I remember that earlier that day, I had found an empty classroom and cried with heaving shoulders into my hands. I remember feeling alone, and small, and mistaken.

And I remember wondering, on that fifth day of medical school, if I would make it as far as February. If I would still be a medical student when the time came for the third dose of that blasted hepatitis B booster.

I never understood how I could succinctly answer the question, "How is medical school going?" It is inevitable that people ask, but whenever posed with this question, I always mentally react with sarcastic commentary. "How is medical school going? Well here, let me give you a genuine, concise answer in one sentence and less than 43.7 seconds."

I am continually stuck when posed with this inquiry. It feels disingenuous to use the noncommittal, easy stock answer that's void of any real substance, but the real one is too winding and whiny to offer up casually.

The truth? The transition to medical school has been incredibly hard for me. I am still unsure if this is where I want to be.

I feel separated from the disciplines I was, and am, incredibly passionate about. I no longer get excited for class the way I did when I was in college taking seminars on racial politics, the construction of scientific knowledge, gender fluidity and medical anthropology. I miss reading ideas and synthesizing my own. I feel uninvested in our material — the science of it feels so detached from the politics and realities of the world. I miss books and discussion and critique; I miss critically questioning what is presented as fact. I think our preclinical education often misses the bigger picture, forgets how medical authority operates, leaves little room to work though the impossible questions of ethics and context and humanity. I am frustrated with a curriculum that relies so heavily on the biomedical framework. I often feel shabby and insecure in all sorts of academic and social ways. I constantly feel that dimensions of my individuality are being flattened by the demands of assessments third and fourth years tell me do not matter anyway.

This curriculum feels displaced from what I pictured a career in medicine would look like. Especially in these preclinical years, our schooling is at once directly tied to becoming a physician, and yet so separated from doctoring. There are also times, scary times, when I realize I have no idea what this career will actually look like as a real profession — that I do not indeed know what I am working towards. People tell me I will have to wait for the wards to know. I worry that when I get there, it will not be what I hoped.

It does not help that surveys show 90 percent of physicians wouldn't recommend this profession for their children.

There is also the new, overwhelming cognizance that there is an infinite amount of knowledge and preparation involved in medical training. There is no end. There is no clear point of termination, and as such, it is up to you to decide where to draw the line of academic sufficiency.

We are told to "be your own guide." This is a reminder meant to provide comfort that your decisions will be right for you, but it is also terrifying. Being your own guide, having autonomy with intention, means simultaneously accepting culpability for anything that goes wrong. It is stressful for me to decide, day in day out, how to optimize my work-life balance. I am young and stupid. I don't love trying to make important decisions about my future while I indeed feel young and stupid.

Medical school has been incredibly stressful for me because it constantly backs you into a corner and forces you to figure out what kind of student and person you want to be, all very quickly. It is an encroaching force that I have to remember to actively push back against as it invades larger and larger portions of my mind, my time and my space. It demands that you decide what is important — to decide what parts of your being you will allow to go to the wayside when you have an infinite number of facts to memorize, an infinite number of ways you "should be" advancing your career. It asks you to balance personal desire and need with the looming pressure of accepting responsibility for the well-being of others. I think oftentimes, this pressure forces us to strip ourselves of the little luxuries that contribute so much more to our identity than the term "medical student." We embrace this title with arms weighed down by books and expectation, and in doing so, we often lose others. We are runners and singers, readers and writers, painters, dreamers, and significant others. But when there are infinite facts to learn, there is less time to run and sing, fewer hours to read and write, diminished capacity to paint and dream and love.

And then there is also this point of guilt: How dare I sit here and criticize and complain about an incredible opportunity that people quite literally dream about. How do I negotiate the idea of finding difficulty in this experience while remaining humble and grateful for the privilege afforded to me by this institution? It also seems useless to worry about having too little time, when I am told over and over that I will never again have the freedom first year allows.

A dear friend recently told me that she thought I was brave for voicing my doubts about medical school openly. This shocked me. I hadn't realized that it was something worth hiding.

Looking back, I suppose I felt early on that there was some shame attached to my doubt. I realize, now, that this notion is toxic, and only served to deepen loneliness and isolation in a place that does not necessarily need to feel lonely and isolated.

Few people are absent doubt in medical school. As I've been more open with my insecurity, I've found more support, more normalcy, and more validation in my beliefs and fears. I've found people who feel the same. These are people I cherish, am indebted to, and care for deeply. I am grateful for the amazing community of peers I have found in my time in medical school — Providence and beyond.

As difficult a transition as matriculating to medical school has been, as much as my doubts are still present, I look back on the fall of 2014 with a lot of joy. Indeed, there were soaring levels of insecurity, creeping levels of worthlessness, and feelings of displacement, but as a whole, my first semester of medical school feels light instead of dark. It is a good place to be, even if I am unsure it is the right place to be.

This is not a well-articulated piece. I have tried to edit sparsely because I don't think this message needs to be sterilized, primped and polished. It certainly has no intention of convincing anyone of anything. It exists purely because I believe validation is one of the most powerful forces in this world.

If you disagree with everything that has been said above, great. I hope this rambly, disjointed reflection has allowed you to feel more situated and confident that medical school is where you are meant to be. If anything I have written resonates with you, spectacular. Know that you are not alone. If you are ever in Providence, come over and drink wine-colored beverages with me on my couch. We can blast Beyonce's "I Was Here" and have some sort of cathartic bonding experience. This is one part of life I will not allow medical school to compromise.

I still wonder what the rest of medical school will hold. What I do know is that when I get punched again by that hepatitis B booster, I will have at least one reason to smile.

I made it to six months.

Cheers to that.

Questions

1. Have you given up other educational pursuits, passions, or hobbies in favor of focusing on medical school? Has the quality of important relationships with friends and family suffered since you enrolled in medical school?

2. What answer do you give to friends or family when asked how medical school is going? Is there an alternate, "real" answer you hold back, and if so, what is it?

3. How open are you with your fellow classmates about the difficulties of medical school? Do you feel pressured to feign confidence?

—Nisha Hariharan

Death and Dying

CMO: Comfort Measures Only, Not Morphine Drip Only

June 8, 2013

Reza Hosseini Ghomi
University of Massachusetts Medical School
Class of 2014

I WAS ON MY INTERNAL medicine clerkship on an inpatient general medicine service at a major academic medical center. It was another long day and our team, from the interns to the attending, was running low on energy. As we entered late afternoon, we received a page for the transfer of a new patient to our service. As the intern read aloud "CMO" — comfort measures only — the team breathed out a sigh of relief and dismissed the transfer from their list of priorities.

I was stunned. This was my first CMO patient, and I wasn't sure why this was such a relief to the team. I soon came to learn what CMO meant for them. CMO meant no diagnostic work to do and no orders to put in, besides a morphine drip. CMO was synonymous with the unofficial permission to ignore the patient. No wonder the team was relieved.

When the patient arrived, she was unable to communicate any of her wishes easily due to severe dementia. She was immediately sedated with boluses of IV morphine every time she stirred in bed. I happened to step in her room as the morphine was wearing off. As I approached the side of her bed and whispered her name, her eyes shot open and she grabbed my wrist while repeating "God help me" over and over again. I called for the nurse and with another bolus of morphine, our patient drifted back to sleep.

I felt sick to my stomach. I did some research and was delighted to find detailed CMO guidelines for our center right on our website. I realized the team had either not known about or had ignored these guidelines. I quickly filled out the form to place the orders recommended by the guidelines. The form itself directed attention to many possible sources of discomfort for patients at the end of life that I had previously been unaware of. For this patient, it had been clear to me that she was uncomfortable. I did not realize until later that part of her discomfort was because she had been written for no food or water for over two days. That certainly didn't sound like comfort measures to me!

Later that day, I felt tremendous relief as I helped the nurse administer the series of orders including eye drops for her bloodshot, dry eyes; lip balm for her dry, cracked lips; an anticholinergic to dry up her airway secretions that were making breathing difficult; a scheduled pain regimen with long-acting medicines to maximize comfort without pain flare-ups; and most of all, a clear liquid diet!

I learned so much from simply following the guidelines already in place. My team was unanimously positive about my proactive approach. Yet, I wondered why my actions were considered exceptional rather than expected.

After seeing my patient drift off to a peaceful sleep, no longer agitated and appearing much more comfortable, I contacted the author of the guidelines, a palliative care physician at my hospital. I spoke to the palliative care physician that same evening just upstairs from where my patient lay sleeping. She explained that although the guidelines were distributed to all caretakers, more often than not, they remained unused. In her many years of experience as a palliative care physician, she has observed that CMO is often translated practically as morphine drip only. She felt the hospital needed to improve the system for orders for these patients, and I volunteered to help out however I could. I went home late that evening wondering how I could help bring about an effective change.

I eventually met with the hospital's chief quality officer and showed him an informal root cause analysis I had done my best to fill out. This was a valuable tool I had picked up through my work with the Institute for Healthcare Improvement and as a campus leader of their Open School chapter. He guided me through completing my analysis and agreed to give this area more attention once he saw data to support the extent of the problem.

I am currently working with the palliative care physician to compile data to demonstrate the standard of care for patients who are CMO. If we are able to collect this data, the hospital has promised to integrate the CMO guidelines into the electronic medical record. This integration would allow the system to detect a patient that is CMO and prompt their caregivers at the level of order entry to step through each evidence-based guideline when placing their admission orders. This will require each area of comfort to be addressed and promote care to progress beyond a simple morphine drip.

This sort of improvement also represents a deeper underlying culture shift in medicine: one in which we no longer view CMO patients — patients who may be expected to die in the near future — as failures, but rather, as opportunities. It frightens me to think of all the patients who still suffer through their last hours when so many comforts are easily accessible, yet unknown. That night before I left the hospital, I remember seeing my patient eating a popsicle with an ever-so-slight smile tracing her lips. She died that night. I can only hope she was in more comfort and peace than when she arrived on our floor.

Questions

1. As a medical student, what challenges do you think you would person-
    ally encounter when caring for a palliative patient, moving from a cura-
    tive intent to comfort measures only?

2. Have you ever noticed a problem with patient care that you thought
    needed improvement, but felt helpless to do anything as a medical stu-
    dent? Does the author's story challenge that feeling of helplessness?
    What can a medical student do at the individual patient level and at the
    hospital systemic level to make change?

3. What factors need to be considered when helping a family and patient
    choose whether to receive end-of-life care in a hospital, in a hospice
    setting, or at home?

4. How would you approach a conversation with a family when there is
    no longer any benefit to curative intervention for a patient? What things
    would you want to say, and not want to say?

—Chelcie Soroka

From Birth to Death:
A Recollection of the Third Year

July 22, 2013

Chris Meltsakos
New York Medical College
Class of 2014

U PON ENTERING MEDICAL SCHOOL, we all knew that we would have to deal with some difficult diagnoses, emotional situations and even death. In fact, even the earliest portions of our training were centered around a cold, lifeless cadaver that we cut into to learn the intricate anatomy and beauty of the human body.

To a first-year medical student, gross anatomy symbolizes the profound meaning of what it is to embark on the long journey of becoming a physician. When one first picks up that scalpel and sets his or her eyes upon the pale skin, with the pungent odor of formaldehyde filling the room, an image is engraved in his or her mind that sticks with them for a lifetime. With the amount of time that is spent working with one's cadaver, one is bound to wonder about that shell of a person that lays before his or her eyes. One recognizes that this body holds the story of a life once lived, bearing life's scars and the wrinkles of time and gravity. It is most medical students' first real encounter with death beyond the extent of attending a funeral.

Yet, as profound as that first experience with the cadaver may be, there are no books, no lectures, no seminars and no words that prepare us to embark on our third-year clerkships. It is a year that starts out with such excitement and flies by quicker than one can believe, yet during this time period, one sees himself or herself grow and mature more quickly than he or she ever believed possible. This transition from a student to a caregiver does not happen overnight. Sometimes it does not even happen until the third-year clerkships are almost over.

Yet for each of us, this transition occurs. Somehow, all of the initial anxiety and nervousness that floods one's mind on the first day of clinical responsibility seems to fade and is replaced by a feeling of, "Hey, I can do this! And I'm not half bad at it, either!"

274

But what is it *exactly* that that fosters this transition? Well, in my opinion, it is a combination of a number of factors. There is great responsibility put on each of us as we progress through the third year. You are now both a student and clinician trying to balance enough patient care with reading and doing well on exams. It is a year in which one feels overwhelmed, overworked and utterly stressed out on many occasions, but somehow each period of stress or anxiety is offset by wonderful memories and experiences gained from both our peers, whom work closely beside us, as well as the individuals that probably teach us the most, our patients.

My third year began with my pediatric rotation. I did not know what to expect, except that I knew that I was not interested in pursuing a career in pediatrics. As the rotation went by, I saw everything from babies seizing from herpes encephalitis to children bedridden and bald battling acute lymphoblastic leukemia.

There was one patient who changed my life forever: an adolescent girl, who was in a head-on motor vehicle accident, sustaining bilateral femur fractures, a radius fracture and pelvic fracture. But more importantly, this was a little girl who watched her mother take her last breath at the scene of the accident. From the first day she was on the floors as my patient, we had an unspoken bond. I stayed many late evenings in the hospital helping to ease her worries and concerns and simply talking to her about anything that comforted her. It was not only a moving experience, but also an emotionally trying experience. On the one hand, it was amazing to see this littler girl improve and get better. On the other hand, my heart was filled with such pain and sorrow watching her cry and tell me about the relationship she had with her mother.

That is when I learned one of my biggest life lessons: the hardest question that a patient will ever ask a physician does not involve the mechanism of action of a drug or the pathophysiology of their condition. Rather, it is the question, "Why?" Whether they say, "Why me?" or "Why my mom, dad, sister, brother, etcetera?" This question is the hardest question to both answer and wrap one's mind around.

As my third year progressed, I saw teary-eyed families surrounding comatose patients as we "pulled the plug." On an overnight call, I had my hands deep inside of an abdomen assisting with a ruptured aneurysm, when the patient expired in front of us. I helped to complete bowel resections and to remove tumors. I delivered babies and saw babies die before they could even experience an hour on this earth. I watched a 48-year-old mother of three with pulmonary adenocarcinoma take her last breath in front of her family as they cried verses from the Bible. For every third-year medical student, the list of life-changing experiences is expansive, with each person finding strength and meaning in different connections that we make or lose.

My third year ended with my internal medicine clerkship — one of the most difficult clinical experiences of my career. We had just admitted a 74-year-old male who was complaining of dyspnea and generalized weakness. Several months earlier he had been told that the B-cell lymphoma that he had been receiving treatment for was in remission. However, six weeks later when he came in for a routine PET scan follow-up, his oncologist found that the tumor had recurred and was now the size of a small grapefruit. We hospitalized him for a congestive heart failure exacerbation, giving him the usual Lasix and contacting his oncologist to visit him in the hospital to administer his chemotherapy regimen.

The patient's oncologist asked me to assist him in relaying to the patient that, despite his chemotherapy, he was most likely going to pass away within the next year. Entering the room with one of the oncology nurses, we explained to the patient that his recurrent cancer was not only aggressive, but also that his comorbidities put him at further risk. If his cancer didn't kill him within that year, one of the other issues could.

First there were a few seconds of painful silence. Then, he asked the nurse some questions about his chemotherapy before asking if he could just talk to me. My heart, having already sank from the initial difficulty of watching a person respond to being told that he only had a year left to live, felt like it was in my feet. I was nervous, scared, sad and wondered, "Why would he want to talk to me?"

I sat down on the patient's bed beside him, as I always did each morning when I rounded on him and said, "I know that this must be hard. I can't imagine what you're going through, but I just want you to know that we are all here to help you every step of the way." That's when he said to me, "You know what, doc? I'm not even scared ... How am I not scared? I'm about to face God and I'm not scared? Do you think I should ask for forgiveness now? How do I prepare myself to die?"

I paused for a moment to collect my thoughts. Slowly, trying to spit my thoughts out, I began telling him that it is normal for people to be numb at first. I tried to address his questions about facing God by telling him that we each have our own connection with the creator we choose to believe in and that he needs to follow what is in his heart to bring him the most comfort. He then proceeded to say, "Well, doc, what do you think it's like, you know ... right before you die?"

Stunned, I took a moment, and then responded, "Well, I suppose I don't know. I mean I honestly don't know. I don't think anyone could tell you that, which is why it's such a scary thought."

We continued this conversation for over an hour talking about both life and mortality and how he could tell his family members. Over the next four days I spent about an hour with him each day, talking about anything that was on his mind. Some days were tearful and difficult, and other days were a bit more lighthearted. One day we talked about whatever food was being featured on the Food Network.

When the patient was ready for discharge, he gave me a big hug and said, "Doc, you're my savior. Thanks for talking to me for all of these hours. I'd have gone crazy otherwise. I know ... I won't probably see you again before I die, but ... I'll watch from up there." He pointed up towards the ceiling. "Good luck with your career. You'll be great."

There is nothing to prepare a medical student for the experiences of third year. One will laugh, cry, feel overwhelmed and stressed. One will feel pride, awe and happiness. Maybe more importantly, though, one will witness the full circle of life from birth to death. The beauty of life and the human body make it a true privilege to be a part of this field. These experiences not only change us as people, but they help shape us into the physicians that we will become. In the words of Sir William Osler: "He who studies medicine without books sails an uncharted sea, but he who studies medicine without patients does not go to sea at all."

Questions

1. An underlying theme in this narrative is the experience of death. Reflect on the experience of death in your own life, whether personal or with a patient. Where did you find strength and meaning in the experience? How will this experience help you in your care of patients at the end of life?

2. In this narrative, the author confronts the question of "Why me?" in regards to the patients he has seen "from birth to death." Have you ever confronted this question in medical school with your patients? If so, how did you interact with your patient, and how did you reconcile the question in your own mind? If not, how will you plan on reconciling your feelings when you are faced with this question?

3. As medical students, we have the privilege of time — more time to spend with patients than any other member of the care team, just as the author did in this narrative. Reflect on a patient you spent "extra" time with and discuss how it affected the patient and how it affected you.

4. What challenges did you experience or do you foresee in the transition "from student to caregiver" during third year? To you, what is a caregiver and what duties does this position entail? How can medical students nurture their inner caregiver?

—Chris Deans

The Inevitable

September 29, 2013

Punita Shroff
New York Institute of Technology College of Osteopathic Medicine
Class of 2014

I WATCHED THE HOSPITAL room in its trickling display of lights — infusions, a ventilator and a monitor with its unrelenting beeping noises. This is what I had come to know of the intensive care unit. As doctors, we are told that we must live and work detached from our patients because emotions can cloud our judgment. But it is difficult to separate emotions when a patient who lies in a bed could be someone's mother, someone's wife or someone's daughter.

I expected the ICU to be a miraculous saving zone. Perhaps it was my naïveté, or perhaps it was the past few weeks I had spent immersed in episodes of medical television shows. "People can be saved," I thought optimistically.

Then it happened suddenly. Admission after admission, death became the status quo. There was no saving here, only prolonging the inevitable. "People come to floor six and seven to go to heaven" became a common phrase echoed daily by the house staff. I scoffed at their words the first few days. Then as the days passed by, I was surprised at the almost obvious revelation.

Not every person in the ICU came to die. Some came to fight with vengeance. But then the natural took over. I remember the sassy spirit of Mrs. C. She came in for one issue, and suddenly her course became a slippery slope. She was eventually intubated, grew sicker and went into septic shock. I was in denial about her prognosis, even though the physicians all said she was going to die. Mrs. C's daughter had tears in her eyes, knowing that it was time. But I held on to hope.

It was only six months ago I sat at the bedside of my gravely ill mother. She survived. I was hoping Mrs. C would be the same. But a day before my rotation ended, Mrs. C passed away. I thought I would cry. I thought that this would be it for me, but instead I just felt the pit of my stomach ache momentarily. After four weeks, I had become immune to death. And in all truthfulness, that saddened me. I reminded myself of the sassy spirit of Mrs. C and her humorous outlook on life in spite of her dire circumstances. She gave me a sense of perspective. Even though we cannot save everyone, we try our hardest, we do the best we can, and the rest is out of our hands.

—

Editor's note: The following addendum to this narrative was written by the author in February 2016.

I wrote this article as a bright-eyed medical student beginning her fourth year clinical rotations. Many of us walk into this profession hoping to be healers, curing patients of ailments and ultimately, saving lives. The art of dying was a hard concept for me back then, and still is for me as a second-year resident. But I have learned that end-of-life care discussions are so important not only to the patient, but to the families and the providers involved.

I know this first-hand. At the time this article was written, my mother experienced numerous health challenges. Her health continued to deteriorate. She was in and out of ICUs with respiratory failure, infections, kidney failure and yet each time she survived. Although she survived, with each insult she became weaker. She was then blessed with a liver transplant, giving her a second chance at life. Unfortunately, this was not enough to keep her alive.

In an ironic twist of fate, my mother passed away in the seventh floor ICU like Mrs. C. In some ways, I connected to Mrs. C's story because it mirrored the mother-daughter relationship I shared. I saw my mother in Mrs. C and it was why many times over the past few years, I remember my patient's face and laughter. It also made me so grateful for the time I had with my mother.

The weeks prior to my mother's passing, we spoke of end-of-life care as a family. We spoke of hospice and we spoke of bringing her home, both of which we were unable to accomplish. I was lucky enough to have a last conversation with my mother, which many families like Mrs. C's never get the chance to have. She wanted me to live happily, and I didn't understand at the time, but my mother was more at peace with her prognosis than I was. She knew and she was ready.

In my grief, I lost sight of my purpose in medicine. But these stories, and the many stories thereafter are all important. They help shape our experiences and provide the framework for our future. Through the process of loss, I began to heal and understand more.

I am thankful for what my mother's journey taught me and the joy she received knowing I was helping others that faced similar obstacles. I learned about the uncertainty of death; for many weeks I laid awake wondering how or when my mother would go. It was the palliative team who worked with us to ease our fears and to make her comfortable. I also learned about difficult conversations, dying and the options available to the terminally ill.

I also learned about grief in its most acute form, and how to help myself (and indirectly others) through loss. Lastly, I learned the strength of moving forward because that is what my mother wanted for me, and as doctors, death is inevitable — what matters is how we choose to deal with it.

Questions

1. How can acceptance of the inevitable help you care for your patients? What are the potential downsides of fighting the inevitable? What toll can this take on the patient, his or her family, and you?

2. Reflect on your first experience with the death of a patient. How has that experience impacted the care you deliver to patients? If you have not yet experienced the death of a patient, how will you prepare yourself for this inevitability?

3. The author wrote an addendum to this narrative about the death of her mother and its parallel to her experience with Mrs. C. Have you ever had a patient who reminded you of a personal or family situation? Did that parallel affect your care of the patient, either in a positive or a negative way?

4. The author submitted this addendum to help her process her immense loss. Do you find catharsis in reading the narratives of others? In writing narratives for others? If yes, why do you think medical students find catharsis in these activities? If not, are there other methods that you believe would better help medical students cope with these feelings?

—Joe Ladowski

Life Song

October 14, 2013

Sophia Tolliver
Ohio State University College of Medicine
Class of 2015

In the key of crunching cartilage,
embedded in a melody of broken hips,
wrapped in a base line of nuts and bolts,
metal syncopated to eruptions
of pain up steep and narrow stairs,
grey and receding memories line
the corridor of this old house.
it and I, we still remember
the creaking of painful harmonies,
storms approaching and penetrating
these walls from the inside out,
we breathe an asthmatic crescendo
in time with the wind and the rain,
in search of the day's weary dusk,
breaking silence, rusty joints fall
down, clanking like jazz riffs...
listen closely to the baa-buh-bum, baa-buh-bum
of a heart struggling to keep pace with a
life song still alive in soft vertebrae and joints,
eroded, worn, and rhythmically crying out in
slowing echoes to the cacophony of our own mortality.

Questions

1. In this poem, the author compares the human body to an old house, with its aging sounds a "cacophony of our own mortality." In what ways is this analogy fitting, and in what ways is it not? Have patients ever described or treated their bodies like aging machines? How might this affect their health, and how might this affect how we treat them?

2. An underlying theme in this poem is the inevitability of aging and death. Have you faced your own mortality while in medical school? What situation or experience made you feel this way, and how did you cope with it?

3. What are the different ways in which the author uses sound to describe the machinery of the human body? Why might it be important to describe the human body to patients in these machine-oriented terms?

4. The description of pain in this poem is vivid. Can you tease out whether this pain is emotional or physical?

—Theresa Yang

False Hope? The Story of Mr. R

October 26, 2013

Faryal Osman
George Washington University School of Medicine
Class of 2014

A S MEDICAL STUDENTS AND soon-to-be future physicians, we are taught to be hopeful when it comes to our patients. We smile; we comfort. We tell patients to put their trust in us because we believe we can cure them. We not only heal with our hands, but also with our words — reassuring when there is doubt, bearing a beacon of light when there is darkness. But what happens when that hope fails to illuminate, and our hands cannot heal?

When I met Mr. R during the first day of my medicine rotation, I never thought he would actually pass away during that hospital stay. I thought that I, along with the residents and attending at our well-regarded institution, could cure him — after all, he presented with a simple pneumonia. He was otherwise healthy, and his prognosis looked good.

I found out Mr. R passed away during our hospital's monthly morbidity and mortality (M&M) conference. I didn't really know Mr. R. After all, I wasn't involved with his care in the ICU, but I was shocked. Mr. R wasn't supposed to die. He didn't even look that sick when my team and I admitted him from the emergency department — he just had a simple pneumonia, not terribly uncommon in an elderly man of 72.

Unbeknownst to me and the rest of our general medicine team, after we had left for the night, Mr. R was then taken to the ICU to be started on an insulin drip for his high blood sugars. From then on, his breathing deteriorated, his pneumonia became worse despite aggressive therapy and he was put on a ventilator in the following days and subsequently expired after his family agreed to withdraw care.

But in hindsight, I think Mr. R may have known he was going to die. Tears streamed down his face as I began to gather the history of his symptoms. He kept glancing at his wife for reassurance, unsure about his fate. In the ICU, when I went to visit him, on his first day, he seemed hopeful and nodded excitedly when I told him I would be taking care of him when he got transferred to the floor.

However, Mr. R never made it to the general medicine floor. I gave him something to look forward to that never came to be.

When Mr. R passed away, I couldn't help but blame myself, even if I was only a medical student and not in charge of his direct care. As soon as I figured out Mr. R was being presented at the M&M conference, I blamed myself for telling him that he would be "okay" that night in the emergency department. Why did I give him false hope? Why did I, as a medical student, try to predict his fate? I know I was fulfilling my role as "the upbeat medical student," but I felt guilty for being positive when I learned that the outcome was everything but okay.

At that moment, a hundred thoughts rushed through my mind: I should be more pragmatic and objective; I should be stoic; I should not be cheerful when I do not know the potential outcome of a situation. I should not give false hope.

Reflecting on Mr. R's situation some months later, I realized that if I don't give hope of any sort at all, I feel I have failed at my role as a medical student and health care provider. As medical students, we walk a tight line when it comes to dealing with patients and delivering their respective prognoses. It is our faces that patients see first in the morning, and it is us who they ask about their lab results, what the doctor says about their latest imaging and, most importantly, when they can go home. We do not want to disappoint. We want to give them good news all the time — that their cancers are not detectable, that they won't need surgery again and that they will be home in time for their children's birthdays. I often feel I need to be positive so my patients feel hopeful about their conditions, even when their diseases are unrelenting.

I know that this is naïve, but I somehow think my optimism can help cure them. And even when it doesn't and patients like Mr. R pass away, at least I know that the "false" hope I gave them did not come from a false place.

Questions

1. Although we observe how illness affects our patients, each patient also affects us in return. Is the author's anger toward herself appropriate?

2. "I was fulfilling my role as the 'upbeat medical student.'" We can play many roles that the author describes: optimist, stoic, objective. Which roles have you observed in a clinical setting? Which were the most well-received by the patient?

3. How do you feel about giving hope to a patient with a hopeless condition? Is it appropriate?

—Andy Kadlec

Try Again: Experiencing Failure as a Medical Student

December 19, 2013

Sadhana Rajamoorthi
Georgetown University School of Medicine
Class of 2014

*S*UNDAY, *8 P.M.* What started as valiant efforts of creating new recipes turned out to be embarrassing failures in judgment and common sense. Initially, I thought mixing tofu, some greens and pasta would turn out to be an Asian delicacy, maybe something that I could proudly share with friends and family. But, after adding one spice to another, topping sauce over sauce, I realized that it was over. It was time to call it an end, let the dish cool and graciously throw it away. As if that failure was not enough, I was up against my next enemy: baking "healthy cookies."

The batter felt thick, so I added water; quickly the batter turned from cookie to cake consistency, and so there I was taking out my new cake pan and pouring what used to be cookie batter into it. Of course, as you would expect, the cake baked, hardened to rock, cooled and then found itself with the ashamed "Asian pasta" in the trash can. Life lesson: don't add water to thick dough if you intend on baking it.

I stood there staring at the ruins of what remained from a bad day in the kitchen. I was irritated with myself, my poor decisions and my miscalculated predictions of ingredients. This was not the first time I was cooking or baking, and I just could not understand why things did not come together. Nonetheless, it was time for me to throw in the spoon and spatula and call it a night.

Monday, 8 a.m. Another day on the cardiology consult service. I finished pre-rounding on my patients, just had a few notes to finish. "We're doing the right and left heart caths on Ms. J around 9 a.m., which you may want to join us for," the fellow offered to me. This was my opportunity to stand behind a glass window and watch a catheter be passed into the femoral vein until we could finally visualize the beating heart in all of its beauty and grandiosity.

As I tiredly sulk into the cath lab, I hear the attending and patient laughing. "Your blood pressures have been consistently soft during your hospitalization, so complete sedation is not an option and any level of sedation would have to be carefully monitored," the attending explained.

The patient laughed it off by responding, "Well, I hope I don't feel too much!"

The site was prepped, and the right heart cath procedure began and then concluded within 20 minutes. "Everything is fine here. We've finished the right portion, now going to move to the left," the physician explained.

"And everything is fine up here, Doctor! I wish I was more out for this procedure, but I'm doing fine," the patient jokingly responded.

Then suddenly, within a blink of an eye the patient's chest began heaving and her extremities flailing. The monitor quickly transitioned from normal sinus rhythm to a flat line. The fellow stepped back, and the attending stepped forward to begin chest compressions and yelled, "Call a code!"

The code team arrived, and within a few minutes the small cath lab became the scene of sheer chaos. It was an army of 11 medical professionals consisting of an attending, residents, nurses and technicians, who stormed in with this focused intensity projecting from their scrunched, serious faces. The attending on the code team quickly refocused everyone and gathered information on what had already been done. I stood in the back, providing information from the patient's chart when asked. So far, chest compressions were started, one dose of epinephrine was administered and the defibrillator was charged and ready to go.

"All clear!" yelled the resident. A shock was delivered and compressions were resumed, but the monitor persistently showed a flat line. The guided execution of the ACLS steps continued, and the attendings began discussing causes of the patient's rapid downfall. The conclusion: most likely anaphylactic shock secondary to intravenous dye.

After nearly 60 minutes of resuscitative efforts, time of death was called, and the code team left the cath lab. As they walked out seemingly undisturbed by the demise of our patient, they discussed who they were going to round on next, dinner plans and funny stories of family situations. I wondered what their thought processes were; they didn't seem fazed at all. For that matter, I was pretty sure that my failed efforts at cooking and baking the previous night caused me more distress than their demeanors showed after the death of a human being. Was it years of experience and the desensitization that comes along with it? Was it the acquired skill of hiding your feelings that medical professionals are so well trained at? Was it the experience of distancing yourself from situations that are technically not in your control? Whatever it was, I knew that I was handling it much differently. After all, this was my first experience in a code amongst some of the most seasoned, experienced medical professionals.

I stood there holding the chart open to the page of family contacts which read, "Daughter: Call cell phone number." The cardiology attending looked at me as I handed over the chart. I could see the disappointment and frustration in his eyes. The cath lab was his comfort area where for years he performed hundreds of catheterization procedures. But, it was now the site of an unfortunate passing of a life, an incident that he may never forget every time he steps into that cath lab. I imagined that he was asking the same questions I asked myself the night before during my baking failure: This wasn't my first time, so what could have happened? Why did this happen? Where did I go wrong?

The major difference was I was dealing with failed cookie batter, and my attending was dealing with a human's life and the daunting responsibility of calling family members. I walked over to the patient. Her body appeared exhausted after that hour of resuscitative efforts, her eyes were closed and the expression on her face was serene. My disappointment over cookie batter seemed so miniscule. On a larger scale, my disappointment over a few poor exam scores, the frustration over those long days during our clinical years, the bitterness over studying my youth years away in medical school were all insubstantial in front of what was lost that morning: a life that used to have love, happiness, family and friends.

As we walked out of the cath lab feeling defeated with our heads hanging down, the second year resident turned to me and asked, "So, do you have any questions?" I assumed he was asking me about the catheterization process or the steps of the ACLS protocol, all of which seemed irrelevant to me in that moment.

I simply shook my head, "No," and continued to walk in silence. I knew that at that moment I needed to reflect; reflect on how transient and unexpected life and death can be, see life in a different perspective and appreciate what I have. Those moments of reflection seemed the best way to honor the patient's life, and keep me sane.

Medical school many times feels like a race to the finish line; who can get to the end first with the most knowledge and skills acquired after years of relentless hard work. We are taught how to identify disease, how to treat it and how to prevent it. We are not taught, on the other hand, how to personally deal with the unfortunate wrath of human physiology in its deepest and darkest moments: death. I suppose it's a self-learning process. For me, I feel that reflecting and putting our experiences into perspective help us cope and continue to preserve the humanistic aspect of the medical care we deliver. Understanding the why and how is crucial but so is protecting our sanity and the respect we have for our patients in both life and death.

If there is one thing I learned from that day, it is to honor — honor our patients, honor our efforts in making their lives better, honor our profession by never losing hope and honor ourselves by never giving up. That practice of not being so hard on ourselves and continually trying to do better begins with the small things in life.

I went home that evening and stepped into the kitchen to make dinner. It was time to pick up the spoon and spatula I had thrown the previous evening. It was time to try again.

Questions

1. The author poses a variety of hypotheses why the medical team seemed unfazed after the patient passed away. Which hypothesis seems most accurate to you?

2. There are many ways that health care professionals deal with the death of a patient. Are there 'healthy' ways to cope with these deaths?

3. What are the resources available to health care providers after the death of a patient? What resources are available to students at your institution?

—Sanjay Salgado

Stars, Dollar Bills, and Other Essentials

October 9, 2014

Morgan Shier
Ross University School of Medicine
Class of 2016

M S. MILLER IS A fading star. At first glance, I begin painting an elaborate picture in my head of Ms. Miller in her brilliant shining glory. Young. Stubborn. Beautiful. Loved. I have no way of knowing if these things are true, but in my head I must believe them because it's just way too sad to accept the truth. Old. Inert. Defeated. Wrinkled. Alone.

Ms. Miller was brought to the ER from her nursing home because she was having trouble breathing. When I greet her, she holds onto her breathing mask with one hand, her eyes focused on something infinite and far away. I quickly learn that she cannot communicate with words, so I begin a physical exam. Normocephalic, atraumatic, signs of respiratory distress. Although she appears lethargic, I sense that she is acutely aware of person, place and time. She is Ms. Miller. She is in a hospital, and it's the end of time.

Her pupils reveal cloudy lenses and constrict slowly to the light that I shine in them. She's thin. She's using extra muscles to breathe. I examine her round abdomen. Her legs are swollen, but I can still feel a pulse in both of her feet. I check her arms to make sure her IV is still in place. In her right hand she is clutching something. She's holding on to it so tight that her long nails have dug into her the palm of her hand. I unfold her fingers one by one. She is clutching a rosary and three one-dollar bills.

Initially I don't understand, but then suddenly I do. She's armed for the afterlife. I let go of her fingers and they snap shut around her possessions. She met my gaze and silently pleaded to keep them.

I walk away. I present the case to the attending. We obtain a chest x-ray, a full set of labs, and call the nursing home to obtain a more complete medical history. Ms. Miller is admitted to the hospital but not to the ICU because, per a piece of paper, we cannot resuscitate her if she should come crashing down. Covered in snuggly white blankets, her fingers tightly coiled over her dollar bills and rosary, she disappears through the double doors of the ER in a flash of dazzling light. Really, she was just wheeled to the inpatient ward upstairs, but my imagination clearly gets the best of me sometimes.

On the train home after work, I remember that when my grandma died, my family made sure to bury her with the same three things she always carried in her purse: tissue, gum and some one-dollar bills. I imagine my grandma carefully choosing these items in life and how they might suit her in death. The dollars stump me because in my version of heaven, everything is free.

I hear the conductor announce my stop. I step out of the train and onto the street. It's cold and cloudy. I complain to myself that it's impossible to see the stars. I know they are nearby though, some bright and some fading away. I know that in my career as a doctor I will meet many Ms. Millers, many fading stars, and someday I will fade away myself. Until then, I will try to live as pulsating life as possible, knowing that I will only need to save a few dollars to take with me in the very end.

Questions

1. What essentials would you take with you into the afterlife?

2. What can medical students do to ensure high-quality care for patients such as Ms. Miller?

3. After encountering "many Ms. Millers," how do you think your response to such patients will change?

4. What are some strategies health care professionals can use to maintain empathy when faced with an actively dying patient?

—Daniel Coleman

Breeze

February 17, 2015

Jennifer Tsai
Warren Alpert Medical School of Brown University
Class of 2018

A WOMAN ONCE TOLD me that babies cry at the slightest breeze because that is the greatest level of discomfort that they have yet experienced in their short lives.

It is a reminder that we can persevere through life's tribulations. That we grow from adversity. That new challenges make past trials smaller.

That this, too, shall pass.

I suppose then, it is a testament to our growth that we no longer cry from warm baths, cooing strangers or scratchy socks. It is uplifting to think that wisps of wind, as innocuous as they are today, were once overwhelmingly strange and violent.

My first experience wearing my short white coat began in a conference room filled with hospitalists awaiting a Morbidity and Mortality discussion. As a first-year medical student, I have not yet become accustomed to the white coat perched atop my shoulders or hooked over my arm. It is still a costume I am scared to don, a pair of big-girl shoes I do not yet feel I can fill — a uniform with too great an authority. My short coat is starchy from inexperience, weighed down by patient checklists, first year flashcards and insecurity. The stethoscope still feels foreign, another accessory that finishes an unwitting costume. I have not grown accustomed to these things, but perhaps with time I will wear them with greater and greater ease until they, like the wind, become nothing but a second thought.

The session opens with a clear objective: "How to understand medico-legal aspects of discharge process and physician liability" — a case study discussing the procedural complications in patients who seek discharge against medical advice. The presenter flows efficiently through the patient history, tongue sliding effortlessly across terms like "ascites," "hematochezia," "hematemesis" and "dyspneic," which are still bulky and encumbered in my mouth and mind. She swiftly recounts the case history of her patient, running through her symptoms, lab results and treatment plan. I am forcibly reminded of how new I am to this journey. The inadequacy creeps.

The conversation shifts to the difficulties of discharge against medical advice, the complicated balance between patient autonomy and physician responsibility. Guiding the conversation is the story of a 59-year-old woman, an anonymous placeholder used to invite the scrutiny and education of physicians. She is a cardboard cutout, a hypothetical patient who left the hospital against recommendation, only to be found unconscious several hours later by her son.

"Time of death 3:25 p.m. called by ED attending."

Stop.

I scramble to flip the presenter's handout back, back, back. There, several slides previous, is a simple chart annotation that suddenly washes other thoughts away.

"Patient wants to go home, her daughter is getting married tomorrow, anxious to leave immediately."

Stop.

My care for the current discussion on discharge procedure and protection against legal retribution is obliterated.

"Time of death 3:25 p.m. called by ED attending."

This woman died on her daughter's wedding day.

My mind is assaulted with pictures of someone else's nightmare. I see a nameless bride wearing a crumpled expression and a pristine silk wedding gown shouting after a retreating gurney, a fiancé thrust too soon into his beloved's unending pain, a harbor of bridesmaids sobbing into bouquets meant to predict a happy future. I think of the confusion. The panic. The heartbreak. The grief.

How did they tell her?

Stop.

Nobody stops.

There is no change to the pace of the presentation. No hiccup in delivery. It continues with a perfect academic examination on the technical difference between "competence" and "decision-making capacity" — a utilitarian departure into semantics amidst a story of a broken family. I have no poeticism to describe this. I am drowning in unforgiving waters yet the conversation stays still and smooth. I am unsure if practice has made these physicians impervious to these assaulting emotions, or if they are merely better at tempering themselves. They pick at their fingernails, refresh their email, check their pagers. Those who remain rapt stay baited with the promise of legal navigation, while I stand trapped by a net of growing distress. Sorrow blooms in the back of my eyes.

This woman died on her daughter's wedding day.

Can you imagine?

Stop.

The idea that many of our most poignant discomforts will one day become peripheral events of the past has given me comfort as I move through life. The obstacles that seemed so insurmountable are now life experiences that I met and passed along the way. The exams that felt impossible, the lover who caused calamity, the rejection letters bearing crushed dreams — these are challenges that felt overwhelming at a time when we didn't have the skills, maturity, and foresight we have now. It is easy to look back and chuckle at how heavy we thought our burdens were. The idea that discomfort is oftentimes temporary and fleeting has always tempered my worry in the past.

But this is different. Far from comfort, the idea that this career will desensitize me to grief and illness and death and dying terrifies me. The loss of others has always been sharp and acute to my being — I daresay it is one of the reasons why I sought to enter the medical profession.

As we surround ourselves with disease and loss, is it inexplicable that we lose our natural reactions to the grief of others? Do we expand our boundaries of discomfort so far that what was once devastating to hear or to tell will become nothing but routine?

Is this what I am supposed to want?

This idea of babies and breezes is a reminder that experience is life's greatest teacher. That experience will tell you what is worth your tears. Your hurt. Your care.

There is a classmate in my small discussion group who has told me "this whole physician sensitivity thing is way overdone." He says it is not only unnecessary, but in fact potentially harmful. But I think there is a difference between being sensitive and being emotional — between feeling sorrow for a patient and being consumed by it. Yes, the distinction is difficult, but whoever said medicine was easy?

I find value in my grief for others. In a world filled with injustice and ugliness among its beauty and wonder, it is empathy that allows us to connect. While I cannot say whether this empathy is definitively a strength or weakness, it is, wholeheartedly, a part of my individual being that I treasure. And whether it is a product of desensitization or merely a mechanism of survival, I do not want grief to be just

a breeze.

Questions

1. In what ways can a physician's grief or emotions be beneficial to the patient and the patient's family, and why? In what ways can these emotions be harmful?

2. Reflect on an experience that was initially difficult or uncomfortable for you, but later became more commonplace, and affected you less. Why do you think the change in you occurred? Was the learning process automatic, or did it require active work?

3. What are some coping mechanisms and specific strategies that can be used to help strike the balance between feeling grief for patients but not being consumed by those feelings?

—Yuli Zhu

Global Health

N'ap Kenbe / We're Holding On

May 14, 2013

Christopher Hudson
University of Rochester School of Medicine and Dentistry
Class of 2016

L ET'S FACE IT: practicing medicine overseas is pretty sexy. Whether it's images of Angelina Jolie and Clive Owen in Cambodia, young French physicians working with Doctors Without Borders, or Paul Farmer in Russian prisons that make you think of international medicine, it all seems pretty cool. Oh yeah, we all have an altruistic motive in trying to help solve the perennial ills of tropical disease, unnecessary trauma and emergency cesarean sections, but there is something about the look on your friends' faces when you tell them you've been living in a *tukul* for three months saving babies.

It is not inherently wrong to feel this way, but it is inaccurate. For most of you who have spent a significant amount of time overseas working, you realize that the moments of bliss do exist, but fall within a haystack of frustration, loneliness and crushing reality. Somehow, needless death, poverty, guilt and betrayal can do wonders to one's previous romantic idealism.

When I left Haiti in October 2010, eight months after the earthquake and what felt like a decade older, I told myself I would never come back. Two weeks from now, I will be going back for the fourth time. The picture I painted in the previous paragraphs seems like a pretty dramatic dichotomy and, while it can be harsh, there is a real pleasure in the life you live as an expatriate in such a troubled and beautiful place.

Previously, I was an aid worker managing internally displaced persons camps in the earthquake-affected zone. This time I will be a medical student in rural Borgne, Haiti. As I prepare for my trip, I find myself wrestling with a lot of the same questions I had on my first big excursion as a Peace Corps Volunteer in South Africa years ago: Where and how can I be most of use? Is this escapade vain or humanist? Is there anything I can really achieve in two months?

As a first-year medical student, I know as much about a patient as I do about cars — I've spent some time around them, but can't really tell you what's going on. This is why I have decided to structure my visit so I can indulge in the training my Haitian superiors in the medical center will generously allow me on *their* time. I have accepted that I am getting more out of this situation than anyone else (which is why I cringe at the thought of the v-word). Because of this, the director of the organization H.O.P.E. Haiti and I have spoken a lot about my long-term commitment to the project.

H.O.P.E. Haiti has done everything right in its tenure as a community-based organization in rural Haiti over the past 15 years. It has worked hand-in-hand with the ministry of health to refurbish and manage the only hospital in the region, it has piggy-backed onto a peasant movement to structure a community health system, it has been in the country way before Haiti was sexy, and the director general is a Haitian-born anthropologist with an unshakable commitment to the Haitian people.

On the other side of the pond, the organization has been fast overtaken by the 21st century explosion of tech- and business-savvy non-governmental organizations. While it has a deep donor base in the US, the marketing, PR and fundraising machines that characterize so many other international organizations these days is forcing H.O.P.E. to reorganize to meet the needs of the work being done in Haiti.

This is where the new cadre comes in. My responsibility to this organization will exceed pretending I know how to treat cholera and taking pictures with some cute kids. As endeavors in international medicine continue to gain popularity among medical students, residents and physicians, there will be a choice that organizations will be forced to make: helicopter in some surgeons for a few hours and pray that nobody needs real post-operative care, or take the time to build institutions through long-term relationships.

So, as I make moves toward this summer, try to put together some trainings for the local staff and present myself humbly to the health care team as a lowly medical student, I will try to keep the vision of H.O.P.E. in mind.

—

So as I wrap up a great weekend with some old friends, I finally have a minute to reflect on my first few days in Haiti, looking at the past and possibilities for the future.

Being back in Haiti is always a shock to the senses. The second you leave the airport your senses are put on overdrive: the cacophony of cars and people; the hot, wet air; the smell of dust, trash and cane; and of course the mosaic of colored tap-taps, mango trees and vendors. It's been almost a year and a half since I've been back and I couldn't be more excited.

The first thing that struck me was the closure of some very high profile internally displaced persons (IDP) camps. For a number of years following the earthquake, the presence of makeshift camps had been ubiquitous. And, suddenly, a huge amount of them are gone. In their place are tall fences surrounding open land that illustrate the government's fear of ever going back to these semi-permanent settlements.

After the initial emergency phase ended, it became rapidly clear that managing the millions of displaced persons in Port-au-Prince and beyond would be an ominous task. The quagmire of land rights, building materials, vulnerable populations, incentives via humanitarian aid for staying in camps and an utter lack of space put the issue at the top of the list. The solution finally came in the form of payments to families (which followed forced removal) as a way to subsidize rent that would be required once leaving the camp. These payments last for one year, followed by small grants that will be used for initial investments that one day may make families autonomous in rent payment and livelihood. Obviously, the success of this program relies on a variety of factors that might just not work out. The precociousness of this position for many families is far from some theoretical plan drawn up in a boardroom in Geneva; it is a real struggle that may mean the difference between life and death.

As the aid money has all but dried up in the areas hit hardest by the earthquake and once flush with cash, such as Leogane, people are forced to pick up the pieces and find a way to survive. The problem with so much of the international aid spent today is so quintessential of our current society. As John Womack puts it, our culture "changes every real, complicated, painful struggle into a brief sensation of stars, or meteors, gloriously noble or wicked, always somehow erotically intriguing today, dead boring tomorrow."

The same is true with aid, and probably with Haiti. We all love the pictures of helicopters flying in and air-dropping food to desperate people, but these things do little to solve the long-term problems that created the crisis in the first place. And, if you dig a bit deeper and look at the historical relations between our country and theirs, it is increasingly difficult to justify the perennial "we can't solve every problem out there" argument.

So, as young people who do care about health inequities, where can we pitch in? Firstly, we have to give the reins to our Haitian partners. The evaporation of aid post-earthquake is such a telling example of how important it is that institutions, not photo opportunities, are built with our assistance. Once we leave, if our work is to have a real impact, the strategy must be owned by Haitians and built by them.

In practice, how do we do this? Here is an example. Although I will be heading to the other side of the country today to work in the H.O.P.E. hospital, I have to be honest with myself that the work is primarily benefiting me. I am receiving the training and clinical exposure and have little to offer in the way of services. However, before I left Leogane my partners showed me sites where they want to scale up projects they have already started. I may want to be cracking the next drug-resistant strain of tuberculosis, but what my Haitian colleagues are telling me they need is housing and family planning. These are the interventions that are important for their community's long-term survival and economic success.

Housing is a huge issue in Haiti because of the financial hemorrhaging that yearly rent bleeds from a family. This is money that could be used to start a business and grow a fledgling economy like that in Leogane. Indeed, all the real progress I have seen since I have been back is Haitian-led. Three years on, practically no emergency food and shelter items remain, but the small businesses that are sprouting everywhere are significant and offer real hope for the future.

Family planning is a similar need. Many women would prefer to only have three children, but access to quality health care tips the balance in vulnerability that yields families with seven or more children and the resources for their development that just aren't there. Instead, with targeted interventions in family planning, families can manage their resources more efficiently to build a life for themselves and create jobs for the community.

In Haiti, you can't exist without asking questions about how to improve society. Everyone talks about it all the time: from physicians to farmworkers to mototaxi drivers to gangsters. Though I had envisioned being on vacation this past weekend, most of our time was spent looking at and talking about new projects. The changes must be Haitian-led, but we can help.

For now, I will be spending the afternoon catching up on emails and getting ready to take a flight to Cap Haitian and from there I'll take a car to Borgne where the real work will begin. Thanks for staying tuned in.

—

Something had happened. The hospital lies on the main stretch of road before the town of Borgne, right across from the high school, so there is always a lot of activity going on: cars going in and out of the hospital, motorbikes dropping off and picking up students, vendors selling food and cell phone credit. But this was different. The cries were not those typical of school-aged children. Plus, it was already 8 p.m., way past the time the last student had left.

A few days prior, water and sanitation teams had been uncharacteristically meeting late into the night discussing who knows what. I am new to the hospital compound, so I don't always feel comfortable snooping around asking everyone what is going on. But tonight, the wailing was eerily familiar. A 35-year-old woman had just died from cholera.

Ever since the epidemic began on Oct. 13, 2010, nine months after the earthquake, managing this archaic, yet vicious disease has been a massive undertaking, especially given the debilitated-at-best state of public health infrastructure, water and sanitation. Despite these challenges, the epidemic has been controlled reasonably well by the hospital here, keeping cases to a rare few in the dry season and a half-dozen during the rainy season. Despite the incredible efforts carried out by Alliance Sante Borgne (ASB) — the H.O.P.E.- and Ministry of Health-managed hospital in Borgne — this woman was unable to seek care before dehydration took its toll. Everyone in the compound is visibly distressed. Many take the death as a personal failure.

I have been in Borgne for two weeks now. My days consist of shadowing physicians in a variety of contexts in the morning, while my afternoons are spent relishing the task of converting the hospital records to an electronic system: an endeavor frustrating enough in an industrialized country, verging on insane in a place like this. There are a few other foreigners, helping to work on the transition to e-records in addition to carrying out a pilot study for a potential project tackling heart disease.

The clinic ranges from a traditional hospital setting to a child malnutrition ward, hosting (or providing) prenatal visits, general consults, emergency intake and even a rural clinic a few hours away by foot. As expected, I feel a bit useless snooping around and asking questions in my clumsy Creole, but the attending physicians are incredibly professional and never protest a request by me to shadow. Most have been trained in Cuba at the prestigious Escuela Latinoamericana de Medicina (ELAM). The ELAM offers scholarships to qualified applicants from countries that lack the capacity to train physicians from poor communities, including a small group of American medical students from under-resourced communities. The program began taking Haitian students on about 10 years ago and has had a massive impact on health care access for the population. It has been said than when Thony Voltaire, the young ASB medical director, came back to his hometown as a new physician, he had people lining up to see him. For weeks he carried out consults without rest. Now the hospital staffs seven physicians, five trained in Cuba and two in Haiti.

As a medical student, the clinical exposure I am receiving is at times unbelievable. I remember just finishing our parasitology unit at Rochester this past spring and students bewilderment at the seemingly endless stream of parasites most had never heard of. Some asked why we had to learn about topics never seen in the United States. Similar questions were raised when learning about tuberculosis and cholera.

On my fourth day in Borgne, I was able to visit one of the rural clinics and followed one of the family physicians doing consults. A young woman and small child came in next. One sentence came out of the mother's mouth. The physician turns to me and says, "TB." I couldn't believe it. The child looked thin, but nothing more dramatic than anyone else I had seen. Then I listened to his lungs and it sounded like crushing tin foil. After a few more questions the child started coughing and the mother's small tissue couldn't manage to capture all the blood that came out. I was floored.

You can read all you want about how devastating a disease like tuberculosis can be, but there is a moment when it switches to something real and powerful and terrible and unfair. I have seen two more cases since then and among the next two, the levels of wasting were much more dramatic. The hospital provides the drugs free of charge, but there are so many extraneous factors that prevent individuals and their families from accessing care.

The commune of Borgne is vast and mountainous. It can take hours, and in some cases days to reach a hospital. Small, rural living quarters exacerbate the spread of this airborne pathogen. Observed treatment can be difficult to organize.

For those of you familiar with the history of poverty and health care in Latin America and the developing world, some of this may not be surprising. There are a handful of organizations doing spectacular work managing unmanageable health care issues. Nevertheless, the problem is deeper than that which can be solved by charitable organizations. This of course is not to say that the impact of hospitals such as ASB is anything less than extraordinary. This is a fact to which every individual touched by this hospital will attest. It does, however, beg the question of what will happen to communities of the same size that have little more than an empty room and a transient nurse as their local hospital. Indeed this was what the health system of Borgne looked like 15 years ago.

As future physicians, it is impossible not to ask the questions necessary to heal our patients clinically. When poverty and economic injustice create the conditions necessary for *treatable* diseases such as cholera and tuberculosis to mercilessly take the lives of our patients, we should maintain our responsibility to ask questions, even if the answers are economic or political.

This is important for those of us who believe health is a human right in any place, but it is also important for improving health care in our own country and, at the most cynical level, to prevent the emergence of pathogens that pay little respect to international borders.

As for me, I will try to remain a fly on the wall and check back soon.

—

Pharmacology is over. I sit in my house with the post-test buzz still ringing in my ear amid a rhythmic background of raindrops striking windowsills and cars sliding past outside. I doze, and the rain conjures afternoons in Borgne when the clinic visitors had slowed to a drip after the morning hubbub.

The end of summer happened fast. At times I have to catch myself to remember that I am back in Rochester since the green and damp could fool tired eyes. When I first started doing these trips I had a much harder time coming back, but now I have become more used to it. Strangely enough, a world where cyclones, tropical hamlets and cane fields can be connected to one with cranes and helicopter ambulances by a short flight doesn't seem so weird after all. Or maybe I have just learned to accept the dramatic inequalities that lie across a puddle of water.

My time in Borgne was wonderful. I observed an incredible amount of medicine from a highly capable team of very dedicated individuals. My already solid respect for the capacity of Haitians was again superseded. Not only was I impressed by the ability for these professionals to provide a basic service in the face of incredible obstacles; I was impressed by their ability to provide a stellar one. Being a bystander observing this health care team makes one wonder about the physician's role within this team. The more I visit Haiti and see the slow progress of rebuilding, dogged perseverance and incredible capacity — especially among the ashes of an international 'humanitarian response' generally accepted to have failed miserably — the more I question why, how and if I can be a companion to this country. When you look at it objectively, most of what's wrong with Haiti has come at the hands of those outside it.

Just look at the past few disasters. In the 1990s, free trade policies brokered by the U.S. government ruined Haitian farmers, resulting in the displacement of millions of impoverished Haitians. Many were in Port-au-Prince when the earthquake hit in 2010, increasing the destruction of the disaster. Additionally, an incredibly resilient form of *Vibrio cholerae* brought to Haiti in October 2010 is surmised to have been introduced by United Nations peacekeepers. To this day, they refuse to admit to this fact and share potentially valuable epidemiological data, and they also shrug off any possible compensation to families or the Haitian government for an epidemic that has killed thousands.

From my limited perspective, Haitians, whether they are farmers, teachers, physicians or even government representatives know best when it comes to their own country. We, on the other hand, do not. Physicians can play a role in Haiti, but it must be done with Haitians in the driver's seat. What we *can* offer is pretty clear.

Training is a huge need for physicians in Haiti, especially postgraduate training, and this is something that academic health centers can contribute towards directly. Advocacy is another powerful tool. Modern Haiti's 'republic of NGOs' has taught us is that a patchwork of well-meaning but ultimately unaccountable foreign organizations cannot replace strong, national health care institutions. This means that more funding and technical support should be provided by our government directly to Haitian institutions in place of donating to American nonprofits or doing Rambo-esque surgery missions that do little to provide prenatal care, public health infrastructure and infectious disease management.

This whole reality has been a tough pill to swallow, yet has been made more apparent the more I visit Haiti. I love that country. I love being there, I love the people, I love the rich history and culture and art and music and pride and raw perseverance. However, I may have to accept that my role in Haiti may be different than the one I used to dream of. The beautiful thing about medicine is that if you truly believe it to be a force for good, it should lead you in the right direction. As I start year two in the long trek towards my MD, Haiti has forced me to accept my failings and take stock of my strengths as I consider what type of physician I want to become. It has forced me to ask myself where and how I can best use medicine to improve the lives of others and challenge a system with entrenched inequality.

On my last day at the hospital I was with the attending physician trying to resuscitate a man in his sixties as his pulses slipped away by the minute. It wasn't dramatic or unique in the sense that it was just another person to die from a disease that held a few headlines in 2010 and then was forgotten. Faintly, you could hear a whimper from a six-year-old boy as he hid underneath his bed sheet in the bed next to the old man's. The boy was the last patient left in the cholera treatment center. You could feel the fear in the room.

Why do we make mistakes that cost people their lives, feel sorry about them, and then keep doing the same thing? This is how we have been dealing with Haiti since it became the second independent nation in the Americas. This is how we deal with health care in our own country. Nobody should have to die from a disease that is as easily treatable as cholera. Nobody should be denied access to life-saving health care based on their social class.

As physicians we will have more riding on the decisions we make because we will see the consequences of our action and inaction at an acute level. We will know what poverty and gun violence and sexual violence do to individuals and communities. I am proud to join a cadre whose work is that critical. I just hope we can get it right.

Questions

1. The author mentions his belief that health care is a human right. Do you agree? Why or why not?

2. What do you think stops physicians from questioning the circumstances surrounding the emergence of treatable diseases?

3. Do physicians have a role in the economic and political side of health care? If so, what is it? If not, why not?

4. What is the role of the physician in international health? Do physicians have an obligation to provide care on a global level? Why or why not?

—Melanie Watt

Half of a Year, Halfway Across the World

September 25, 2013

Sadhana Rajamoorthi
Georgetown University School of Medicine
Class of 2014

C *HENNAI, INDIA.*
"How are you feeling?" I asked an elderly woman in Tamil, the local language. She had recently been diagnosed with rheumatic heart disease at the hospital. I struggled to hide my excitement of finally being able to interact with an inpatient after three weeks of waiting for a "TB-free ward."

In the Western world, we quarantine patients with tuberculosis; here they are one of the many patients in the general ward who are seen by doctors and students not wearing face masks. The theory behind this, as was explained to me, is that India has the world's largest TB epidemic, so any single individual is at risk whether he or she is in a hospital or in the grocery store. The only thing anyone can really do besides wear a face mask all the time is to hope that their immune system is strong enough to ward it off. Faith aside, I decided to play it safe and wait for a "TB-free ward."

"I'm feeling better, I do not have pain anymore," she replied in Tamil. I did a thorough physical exam, reviewed her chest x-rays and lab results. I took about 15 minutes to explain all of the results and told her that she is looking a lot better, with all of her imaging and lab results supporting that finding.

I was very excited for her, but she showed no emotion. "Doctor, I've been here too long. My family is struggling without me. Does this mean I can finally go home?" she asked.

"Yes, of course! We are discharging you from the hospital today," I replied.

Her face finally lit up, but it left me feeling very confused. *How could you not want to know about the progress of your disease? Or be excited for the improvement in your health?*

As Dr. Varadarajan and I walked back to the outpatient department, he

307

explained to me, "The patients we see here barely understand their diagnosis, let alone the prognosis or treatment process. The details of their disease just don't matter to them. Most of them come to us at later stages of their disease because they just can't afford to leave their families. They live from meal to meal, and that's all they can focus on."

With that in mind, I learned to cater my questions and explanations towards these situations. But even then, it was impossible to accept the devastating poverty that people face in developing countries.

The next patient I saw that day was a thin young man with a stained towel wrapped around his right foot. He limped into the room barefoot, which is quite common in poverty-stricken areas. The doctor asked the man to remove the towel, and I felt my breakfast travel back up my stomach into my mouth. "Gangrenous" would be an understatement for what we saw. The patient was sent to surgery, and as he limped out, the physician told him, "Don't worry about paying for your services here today. Just use that money to buy yourself shoes. I don't want to see you barefoot ever again."

Over the next few months, I saw everything from tuberculosis (of course, never in direct contact) to malaria to dengue fever to parotitis to thyrotoxicosis. I even saw rare cases, such as Plummer-Vinson syndrome, Tetralogy of Fallot, leprosy and a cribiform plate injury with cerebrospinal fluid rhinorrhea. But, beyond the mind bending cases, I saw something equally as amazing: faith.

There was one instance where I was asked to interpret a chest x-ray for a woman with severe dyspnea. I walked over to the patient to perform a lung exam. She was an elderly, frail woman, sitting hunched over in a wheelchair. I took my stethoscope out of my pocket and placed it on her chest. She placed her hand on my hand that was holding the stethoscope, looked at me with tears in her eyes, and said, "Please don't let me die. You are all God's messengers; I trust you with my life and have all the faith in the world that you won't let me die." The intensity of that situation and the pain I saw in her eyes left me numb. The level of faith she had on her medical team was humbling, but at the same time overwhelming.

Many times, even after a diagnosis was fully described, patients in some parts of India would still ask, "Doctor, am I going to die?" It is not a matter of ignorance, but a preference to trust the physician with that knowledge. These people feel comfortable in leaving the decision-making process completely to their physicians. This is in contrast to the patient-centered model that we see in some of the bigger Indian cities and in the Western world. This system is based on medicine being treated as a team effort, with physicians providing guidance and health care, while patients do their best to stay compliant with their medical regimes.

After nearly half a year in India, I learned that providing medical care to the underserved requires a great amount of trust-building. Skills and knowledge come with dedicated practice and years of experience. However, the ability to connect with people and gain their trust requires patience, respect for every individual, and gratitude for the opportunity we've been given to touch peoples' lives. Rabindranath Tagore, an Indian poet, once said, "I slept and dreamt that life was joy. I awoke and saw that life was service. I acted and behold, service was joy."

I'm sure that we have all experienced one moment where we felt pure joy after making a patient smile, feel better, or helping him or her through a difficult time. I'm sure we can all agree that there is no greater joy than that.

Questions

1. Do you agree with the author's statement at the end? Have you found joy in helping a patient?

2. Why do you think there has been a shift from trusting doctors to make medical decisions to a culture of patient autonomy?

3. The author discusses the need for trust-building when serving underserved populations. Why is trust important in health care? Does it take a long time to build, or is it instantaneous?

4. Is trust harder to build with patients in foreign care settings? Why or why not? Is trust important for all health care interactions?

—Melanie Watt

The Problem With Playing Doctor: A Critique of Student Medical Outreach from Within

December 4, 2013

Shraddha Dalwadi
Texas A&M Health Science Center College of Medicine
Class of 2017

"**I**S THE PAIN SHARP or dull?" I say to the teenaged translator next to me. Rolling her eyes, she quickly mutters something in Spanish to my distressed patient and then relays his response back in English. As she returns to texting on her cell phone, I make the final notes for this patient. Although I have reached the end of an extensive two-page history, I can't help but feel completely unaccomplished. I've been told this is the most important part of forming a diagnosis, yet the unyielding language barrier has caused me to fail to form any sort of trusting relationship with my first patient.

While we wait for the doctor to come to our station, I study my patient. His build is strong, but for the heaves and lifts of his overworked frame. The patient looks up at me, with skin leathered from the Costa Rican sun, and wears a big smile — he is excited to see an American "doctor." His son, wearing a cloth diaper and a mysterious rash, eagerly plays with the other students in my group. I smile back, but only for a moment. I find it difficult to look my patients in the eyes sometimes, fearful that they'll read me for the inexperienced medical student I am.

It isn't until the doctor comes by that the real magic happens. I methodically repeat a summary of my history and, instantly, she can tell this man suffers from chronic, untreated hypertension. She writes a prescription and sends him off to our improvised pharmacy. A student fills his order, and my tired patient faithfully takes his first dose while waiting for his son to be treated.

Five minutes later, I hear commotion coming from the waiting area. The man has fallen unconscious, and his son is screaming in terror next to him. Ten minutes later, the doctor discovers that the pharmacy filled the wrong drug; this man is now fighting to stay alive. Thirty minutes later, he's loaded into an ambulance, and yet an hour later, things are back to normal at our clinic. We're almost glamorously serving these people, taking pictures with their delightful malnourished children, and practicing our sub-par clinical skills.

In our seven days, we never saw the man again. In fact, we never saw any of our patients for a second time. Not one of the 1,427 patients was ever seen for follow-up of their diagnoses. I worry that they did not consider it important to finish the full course of their antibiotic, that their children ate too many sweet gummy vitamins, or that they simply did not see their transient dizziness as the serious medical concern diabetes is.

On my airplane ride back, I couldn't help but wonder: *are we just fooling ourselves?* We hold up our stethoscopes to their skinny bodies in excitement, our unsophisticated ears hear something (anything!), and we call it normal. We are afraid to touch the patient, we cannot even hold a conversation with them, and yet we truly feel that we are helping others. Are we just playing doctors?

I agree that the intentions behind hosting a medical missionary trip are good. However, as the premed and medical students who run these endeavors, we must appreciate how great of a responsibility we are undertaking. Much work needs to be done on our part to make sure the service we provide abroad is of the same caliber of that which we would provide in our own clinics.

Before we step inside the other country, education about the language, clinical skills and culture needed to best serve the area should be customary. Even if we still require translators, imagine how much of a difference simply asking the history in the native language would have on the patient-provider relationship. In addition, native doctors for supervision and establishment of proper follow-up for patients must become protocol. Lastly, an emphasis on public health education must become a priority for these underserved areas, where a month's course of vitamins will not accomplish as much as an informative focus on nutrition and hygiene.

Our purpose is sincere, and sometimes we truly are able to help the febrile child with antibiotics or the middle-aged woman to discover her condition as menopause. Other times, we are walking a tight rope. Focused on serving an abundance of people with very few resources, we may forget that being a medical professional relies on the principle of nonmaleficence. Often, these people see students on mission trips as a reflection of modern medicine itself. If we fail them, they may lose their hope in all doctors. It is imperative that we uphold a high standard during such efforts, not only to show the validity of quality health care, but also to help more than we hurt.

Questions

1. Have you ever gone on a health care-related trip abroad similar to that of the author? What was your motivation in doing so? In retrospect, was the trip worth it? To you? To your patients? To the health workers abroad? To the health workers who traveled with you?

2. Is seven days enough for you to help patients abroad? If yes, was it a significant and sustainable difference? If not, then what is the purpose of traveling abroad in this manner? How can we make these trips more helpful to the providers and to the patients?

3. Have you met a patient who had lost faith in the medical system? What was his or her story? Were you able to help?

—Nisha Pradhan

Perspectives from the Bike:
A Look at an Ecuadorian Hospital

January 23, 2015

Brian Lefchak
Drexel University College of Medicine
Class of 2017

T HE GRAY PICKUP TRUCK rattled along the rocky path, careening back and forth on a steep incline that reached for the snow-capped peak masked by clouds. While tires slid and kicked up trails of dust that diffused into the mist surrounding us, I was still able to catch a glimpse of Chimborazo, a volcanic pyramid of Ecuador, through pockets of clarity in that atmosphere. Soaring at breathtaking elevations of over 20 thousand feet, Chimborazo is a point near the equator where one can be closest to the sun while standing on Earth.

Upon reaching a small plateau somewhere closer to the top, my guide, Galo, helped me suit up with elbow pads, knee pads, a helmet and hat, radio and other protective gear to wear over the four layers of clothing I had come prepared wearing. I looked up into the deafening silence of clouds rolling lifelessly like tumbleweeds across a primordial landscape flattened underneath the might of a glacial throne. Then I pushed the bicycle off and started my way down.

The long and rutted way down stretched out before me through a chilly and otherworldly landscape of lunar gray and dull tan colors, dotted with small shrubs and the occasional pack of wild vicuñas, animals closely related to the llama. I continued downhill on the muddy trail as dusk quickly approached and found myself amidst tiny concrete structures and huts, the houses of rural villages. The homes sat scattered apart from one another along the dirt trail, some windowless and others with crude metal roofs.

On more than one occasion, I was forced to stop for the animals blocking the trail, whether they were cows and sheep roving along to some new undiscovered plots of grass, or llamas staring with curiosity at me, the alien in their habitat. However, the most memorable aspects to this developing scenery were the local inhabitants. In particular, I saw the children of the villages here and there, many appearing to be no older than six or seven years of age. They would come out from the grass nearby or from chasing their wandering livestock to watch, sometimes trying to run alongside the foreigner on a bicycle zooming by and then, just as quickly, disappearing into the evening redness of the horizon.

Fresh in my mind throughout this mountain biking endeavor were the previous two weeks, which I had spent working in the pediatrics ward of a general hospital in Riobamba, Ecuador as part of a medical Spanish immersion program. I thought of the children I interacted with there, the doctors I observed, the differences in culture I questioned, the Spanish I gradually improved, and the continuing discoveries I made regarding the spectrum in which medical care is provided across the globe.

At the risk of oversimplification, the hospital floor where I worked was comparable to a time capsule notion I have of the 1960s or 1970s American hospital, which I admit I have only encountered in films. One would find that the rooms had multiple beds — all rudimentary — occasionally paint-chipped metal frames bereft of electronic position adjustments, and often fully occupied. Nurses, without exception, were dressed in starched uniforms, donning old-fashioned nursing caps on their heads, with male nurses even more noticeably absent than I had reasonably expected. Paper records and forms stood in place of computers and technology. The extent of morning rounding followed by afternoon outpatient work by the same physician demonstrated to me that hospitalists were much less commonplace. Telling above all, however, was the primacy and final authority of the physician in health management, which was in rather glaring opposition to much of the patient-centered care that we, in the United States, are taught in medical education.

It is rarely, if ever appropriate, to point to one single factor in any analysis because there are more often many forces at play. Indeed, many features of what I call this "time capsule" comparison are the result of several factors: Ecuador's economic development, South American cultural differences, my observing a general hospital as opposed to a private insurance facility, the particular region in which the hospital was located, and the fact that it served a wide area of patients, most of whom were indigenous. Despite all I saw in Ecuador, clearly there was much more I had not witnessed or experienced during my limited stay. Nevertheless, the differences stuck out strong to my foreign eyes, whether it was the manner in which iodine was poured over surgical appliances prior to quick procedures, the general weathered appearance of the blue tiles of the ward's hallway dotted with pealing images of cartoon characters, or the traditional, colorful and hand-sewn indigenous clothing that so many of the patient's parents and families wore.

The three most common conditions I saw affecting the children were pneumonia, malnourishment and automobile accident traumas. Pneumonia presented so routinely that patients with infections, no matter how young, were usually the ones in and out the quickest. Malnourishment revealed itself in such cases as a four-month-old boy with kwashiorkor and an indigenous baby with cleft lip whose weight contraindicated surgical repair. We witnessed a significant amount of motor vehicle accident traumas, too. I witnessed two young boys, terrified inside the hospital, suffering from fractures of the humerus as a result of being hit by a car. The worst trauma victim I saw had temporal-parietal fractures, face lesions and secondary left leg immobility which left him initially unable to walk. I still remember the raw panic in the boy's face when he was unable to comply with the doctor's order to raise his leg.

There was a baby with hyperbilirubinemia who was placed under UV light as part of treatment. There was a little girl who had suffered maltreatment and abuse from her mother, whom all of the nurses on the floor promptly seemed to shun. We saw a young boy with tangible hepatomegaly and Hodgkin's lymphoma, multiple patients with HIV infections, a boy with hernia and sepsis, and so forth, some more routine and others more serious. Many of these conditions I was expecting to see at some point back home, while others I now do not know if I will ever see again.

As rewarding as the pediatrics experience was, I also believe that the differences in hospital culture became most apparent within the pediatric setting. For example, during rounds, all visitors, including parents, were required to step-out of the room, an uncomfortable separation for both the parents and their children, who promptly began screaming. Furthermore, I had difficulty understanding what might have been considered normal behavior for medical professionals interacting in the presence of patients. Some personnel seemed more interested in having fun, even making inappropriate jokes in front of their patients, instead of actually talking to and comforting the visibly lonely and frightened children.

Consequently, we did do just that and began talking to the children so that we could not only practice our Spanish, but to hopefully make an inherently frightening setting a little less intense. We also were curious to hear what they thought of the hospital in their own words. Our first attempt was met with confused and guarded expressions, as if the children were wondering why they were being approached by yet another white coat. One of these children was the frightened young boy with a fractured humerus who had arrived at the hospital after being hit by a car. Within just a short span of time, I can recall entering his room to find him sitting up, smiling and waving to me whenever I walked towards the often empty chair next to his bed. I always had the impression, even upon leaving, that some of the residents-in-training at the hospital found the foreigners' patient conversations odd, but frankly I began to not care about that.

In fairness, however, we also observed many heartwarming episodes and recoveries, sincere care and concern demonstrated by the physicians we looked up to, and even the simple, inherent goofiness of doctors and staff playing and interacting with the kids. The boy who had presented with

315

temporal-parietal fractures, panicking because of the earlier condition involving his leg, gradually regained his ability to walk. Over the span of many mornings on rounds, the child, perhaps four feet tall, surrounded by a sea of white coats towering over him, initially stumbling back and forth between his bed and the door, gradually was able to walk the distance as if it were completely normal; the terrible swelling in his eye reduced, and the red lesions across his face quickly began to heal by the time I had left. It was difficult to not be moved by that sight.

The pediatrician I shadowed during external consult genuinely enjoyed his work and cared about his patients. He established a routine that consisted of fist bumps rather than shaking hands. It was evident that instead of treating his patients as checkboxes, this physician showed interest in more than just the child's physical health. He was well-informed and invested in advocacy. In particular, he highlighted the importance of improved instruction and regulation in driving customs in order to prevent the accidents. He emphasized improved sexual education in schools as a means to remedy the division of gender-related conditions that we had also seen in patients. Finally, he called for improved education in nutrition and cooking to prevent the kinds of malnourishment present in poorer rural populations that resulted not so much from the lack of food, but rather from the cultural methods of food preparation.

All of this was on my mind on that last day before leaving Riobamba as I saw the children alongside that dirt trail in the countryside around Chimborazo. In particular, I thought about a little girl who presented to the pediatrician's office only a few days before with a significant heart murmur, a tangible foreboding of what possibly lay ahead. She was of the indigenous population from a rural area. The girl would have to be taken all the way to the capital, Quito, for an echocardiogram to determine her diagnosis as the test was not available for children at the Riobamba hospital. For many of us living comfortably in the developed world or even for those of us with significant struggles, it is difficult to fully appreciate just what something like this meant for these people. The capital was three to four hours away, not to mention the difficulty involved in actually traveling to the hospital for a family with no car. The child would then have to receive the procedure after sitting among the long lines of people in crowded hallways we had seen waiting for an appointment every day for the past two weeks. Uncertain still were the results and implications of the echocardiogram and the number of days this family of very modest means would have to spend in the capital far from home. The child sat there following her examination, calm and at ease with a slight smile and large dark eyes that were unable to see her path ahead. The mother, despite discerning more clearly the inherent implications, also smiled upon looking at her daughter's face. Upon their leaving, the pediatrician shook his head, as if in disappointment that there was nothing else to be done and little else he could say, a feeling far too familiar.

While I may never know what happened to that family, I could not help but think about them and the other patients we had seen, so many of whom had come from the very conditions I found myself unexpectedly witnessing firsthand on the bike trail that stretched out ahead. It made me wonder which of these children, there running alongside llamas and sheep, would have to travel the two hours to the nearest hospital in Riobamba under similar circumstances or which will be unable to acquire the care they needed and deserved. While the hospital experience shed light on our collective shortcomings, it too highlighted the immeasurable impact of individuals devoted to their specialties and the resilience of people willing to sacrifice in ways unimaginable in spite of the odds against them.

Near the snow-capped upper heights of Chimborazo, I was unable to glimpse the summit, and even upon descending, I never was able to see the mountain in its entirety. However, I found myself pleasantly surprised by what I discovered during the descent: the views and sights of the locals in the villages I could not see from either the upper heights of mighty Chimborazo, nor from within the hospital in Riobamba. I never could have anticipated holding the images of that day so vividly in my memory even up to now. The bike trip served to put in perspective for me a journey far larger, an apt reminder of what our focus, motivation and attitude should be along the path we choose in medicine.

And besides, the view of the mountain from the bottom looked better than from the top anyway.

Questions

1. The author uses a simple yet exhilarating bike ride as an allegory to his medical training. What experiences, creative encounters, or athletic pursuits can you use to better understand your training?

2. The author's bike ride is a trigger for his reflections on Ecuador. Do you have triggers for reflecting on your experience in medical school? Do you reflect on a day-to-day basis, or does the "exotic locale" induce a different type of reflection?

3. The contrast between American medicine and that of developing countries can be stark. The author describes economic and cultural etiologies for this contrast. What other possible sources might account for these differences?

4. Medicine is defined by human interactions. The author describes patients that have stayed in his memory since his trip to Ecuador. It is important to have memories like these, brands and tattoos of our past experiences. What do yours look like?

—Brent Bjornsen

An Afternoon with a Swazi Boy

January 27, 2015

Brent Schnipke
Boonshoft School of Medicine at Wright State University
Class of 2018

Mostly, because I don't know
what else to do, I take the hand
of this little boy, different than me
in so many unimportant ways.
His feet are calloused
from the hard red rocks;
my hands are cracked, from overuse
of Purell hand sanitizer.
He sees his world clearly
and knows all about it; I am
so young and inexperienced.
His mother and father are dead.

The only thing darker than his skin
is his prognosis, I think bitterly.
Earlier today I spilled his blood,
just enough
to cover the test strip, enough
to show me the two red lines
I was praying wouldn't
materialize. But they did.
I grip harder than I should
and think about the pain
he feels. How could he not?
But he does not speak of pain;
he is merely intent on kicking
the wadded up paper covered

in packaging tape — a sad excuse
for a soccer ball, to me,
but to him and the others
a source of daily joy.
It bounces erratically,
but the boys have steady feet
to match their steady laughter.
He looks at me. His black lips part
to reveal teeth that are whiter than me,
and his eyes say, *friend!* I give
a final squeeze and he goes off to play.

The little paper test had told me
he was positive, but I needed
an afternoon with him to know
just how much more positive
than me he was.

Questions

1. Think about a time when you had just learned "bad news" about one of your patients. What emotions did you experience? What did you feel when you saw the patient for the first time after learning the bad news?

2. Has there ever been a time when you delivered bad news and were met with a response that you did not expect? How did you react? Why do you think the patient or family reacted in this way?

3. How do you find the "positives" when caring for a patient with a grave diagnosis?

—Aleena Paul

On a Mission

January 28, 2015

Victoria Psomiadis
University of South Florida Morsani College of Medicine
Class of 2017

M Y ARM WAS STILL aching from the yellow fever injection when I saw my first real patient.

Sitting across the table from me was a woman with four children, whose hesitancy towards their foreign doctor mirrored my own. I still wonder sometimes how I ended up in that tiny cinderblock-and-corrugated-metal church in Bolivia, not even finished with my first year of medical school. At the time, I felt frantic. I was convinced I had no skill and no knowledge to help the people who waited patiently in line all day for our little plastic baggies of vitamins and antiparasitics. Less than a week later, when I stepped off the plane and back onto American soil, I felt very differently about my capabilities.

Medical missions are a popular part of medical school culture. Heading off to the Caribbean or South America as a first-year is exciting and a great resume item for residency applications. It makes you feel good about yourself and your clinical skills. Despite the obvious dangers of traveling abroad, many organizations on campuses across the nation make it a key selling point of membership. Spring break, for those lucky souls who are accepted to the team, is an adventure totally beyond any previous experience. For some of us, it is life-changing.

Last week, I sat down with the officer team of the Christian Medical and Dental Association to review applications for our annual trip. Looking over the applications brought back memories of writing my own application: the frenzied preparation, the anticipation, the terror of landing in a country where my solid A's in high school and college Spanish suddenly felt useless. I remembered talking to many of the first years whose applications now were neatly organized across the screen of my laptop, and telling stories of exploring the city while dodging the paint-filled balloons of kids celebrating

Carnival. I found myself excited for the twelve who made the cut, knowing the memory of this trip would subtly shape them, as it had shaped — and still is shaping — me.

I am not the same person I was when I left the States bound for South America last spring. The first-year who got on that plane was tired, sad, and burned-out. After an extremely difficult academic and personal quarter in school, I was starting to doubt that medicine was right for me. I spent most of the long flight worrying that I didn't know enough to do what I needed to do, and that when I got home I'd be calling my parents to give them bad news. However, a small part of me clung to the hope that Bolivia would heal some of the damage.

The things we expected, happened. We saw hundreds of patients in those few days. As I expected, I gained experience in physical exam skills and comfort in patient interaction, confidence in my abilities and knowledge, and a greater appreciation for the quality of medical care I can receive just by walking into the student health clinic. Working in small teams of two students and a translator with only a few upperclassmen and two doctors to fall back on, we learned to recognize and triage chief complaints. My first-year partner and I quickly learned the use of most of our medications, and could explain the dosing regimen of almost every item of our formulary in Spanish without the help of our translator by the end of the week. Since I traveled with a religious organization, I also anticipated the renewal of faith and purpose that comes from constantly praying and reflecting on little moments of the day. I was not disappointed socially, either. The new closeness with my team, some of whom I barely knew beyond a name and a face before the trip, has continued and strengthened as we've moved into our second year. Like many medical students on mission trips, we worked long hours. We'd leave the house early in the morning and stumble back in wrinkled scrubs, but still summoned the energy to play soccer with the locals and stay up late with games.

I don't think, however, that I anticipated how a one-week medical service trip could reignite my passion for medicine and service work, and begin to direct my career path. Since our return, I have seen many of my teammates (and myself) leaning towards primary care. I was interested in providing care to underserved populations before medical school began, but since my trip, it has begun to solidify as the end-goal of my education.

Medical mission work does not have to require vaccinations for tropical diseases, a passport and a warning note on the sink reminding you not to drink the tap water. While there are plenty of organizations that allow practicing physicians to travel abroad and provide care, there are large areas of our own country that can benefit from the same services. There are government-funded programs that require a commitment to practice in a medically underserved area in exchange for tuition payments. Large urban centers have neighborhoods in which health care access is desperately limited, and many of the far-flung rural communities that exist across the nation are dangerously far from hospitals and trauma centers with only a few general practitioners serving to cover large geographic areas. Religious and secular charities fund nonprofit free clinics staffed entirely by volunteer providers. And you need not cross a national border to find patients who need translators to tell you about their shortness of breath.

Medical mission work as a medical student is mind-altering if you let it be. Finding yourself autonomous, useful, and knowledgeable in a difficult clinical setting breeds a confidence that medical students crave. For some, it also feeds a fire we may not have noticed smoldering inside our hearts. These are the students who come back in third and fourth year, and who apply for service positions and residencies in rural and impoverished urban settings. Some of them go on to work for free clinics, to travel with international aid organizations and charities, or to live as missionary doctors in foreign countries.

When I first began meeting with the incoming students this year, I told them both sides of the medical mission story. I told them about the joys of listening to the heartbeat of an unborn child with the mother for the first time, hearing a native Quechua woman call you *doctora*, having a precious little boy and his tiny puppy fall asleep in your arms as you listen to the murmur in his heart. I laughed and nudged my teammates as we recounted the tales of soccer games won and lost, impromptu sing-alongs in the van, the lack of fresh vegetables, and the swollen ankles from travel and a high sodium diet. But interspersed among the laughter were more serious things: the poverty, our nerve-wracking firsthand experience with local medical care, the heart-breaking gratitude of people our limited resources were unable to help, the feelings of guilt, and longing for my narrow bunk in a room with six other women upon my return to the comforts of my own home. Warnings about low-maintenance lifestyle requirements, disguised as jokes about the shower tap that shocked you every morning, were counterbalanced with exultant stories of catching rare diagnoses. I admitted to them that I still find myself homesick for Bolivia, and that if I could, I would gladly return to the humid heat and the mosquitoes and the ramshackle churches that served as temporary clinics for our team.

In telling both sides, I hoped to show them what I learned when I sat down with that first patient and her children: there is selfless service that benefits others, and there is selfish service that benefits the servant. And sometimes, a mixture of both sends you on a mission to discover who you are, what challenges and excites you, and what role you will take in the world.

Questions

1. Why do medical students flock to serve in foreign countries when there are so many medically underserved patients to care for here in the United States?

2. How can traveling medical students ensure that the care and services they provide are sustainable?

3. For medical students who cannot afford, financially or time-wise, to travel internationally, what are some other experiences they might seek to reaffirm their passion for medicine and use their skills altruistically?

4. How does the author's faith and the faith of the Bolivians' she served affect their medical care? Do you think faith makes the physician-patient relationship stronger?

—Brent Schnipke

Feeling Like
a Physician

More Than a Number: The Patient's Story

November 11, 2012

Peter Wingfield
University of Vermont College of Medicine
Class of 2015

T HOUGH I AM CURRENTLY A second year student at University of Vermont, I actually started medical school back in the '80s in an ancient and venerable school in England, granted the royal seal by Henry VIII. Even just twenty-five or so years ago, the nurses still wore uniforms not significantly different from that worn by Florence Nightingale herself, and they kept their heads bowed and eyes demurely averted on ward rounds. I remember that there was never any doubt that "Doctor knew best" and that his word (and I use 'his' advisedly) was beyond question or reproach. He would make his pronouncement and the 'angels' would do his bidding.

After a tortuous journey, I am back in medical school, many years and several thousand miles removed, and I am struck by how different the view of care is now. "Patient-centered care" means doctor as steward but at the helm of an integrated team, encompassing many disciplines and with a goal of understanding the patient's viewpoint as the target of primary designation.

My peculiar, somewhat unique history makes me view things rather differently from most medical students. It makes me very conscious that things are transient, not immutable. What we believe to be true of good practice today may be the focus of ridicule to another generation. So as good stewards we need to be looking for those things that are eternally true and fostering them in our ever-evolving ideas. The practice of medicine will continue to change beyond all possible recognition from where it is now, but that is not new; it has always been the case. If we look carefully to the past, it may help us to understand our future, because some things that were true in Hippocrates' day still hold true now, and these are the ones that are likely to continue to be true in the coming centuries as well. Perhaps for this reason I am repeatedly drawn back to a wonderful quotation from William Osler:

"It is much more important to know what sort of a patient has a disease than what sort of disease a patient has." I believe that this is one truth that is unlikely to change.

We, as a species, are at a time of unprecedented transformation. We are preparing ourselves for a future that no one fully grasps and the world in which we will practice medicine is something of a mystery to us. All that we can confidently say is that it will be different from the one we see around us now. Yet we are educating ourselves largely as we did a hundred years ago. Technology is advancing at exponential speed, and we seem hell-bent on coming up with cleverer and cleverer ways to use the number crunching power that so enchants us. There is a significant risk in this, however. The more we believe that a patient can be reduced to a series of aliquots of data, the more inevitable it is that the digital, silicon-based life forms we are creating will make us obsolete in the care of ourselves and our fellows. We also seem blind to the fact that we will become irrelevant if we compete with them at things they were specifically designed to do better than us, rather than use and embrace them as differentially functioning partners. Is it in anyone's best interest for us to be focusing our attention on skills that will inevitably be done far better by a laptop?

I anthropomorphize the computer in order to illustrate one of our historical Achilles' heels: failing to appropriately value the input from sources outside our own cerebra. We frequently give too much weight to shiny new ideas and are blind to the enduring simple power that comes from observation of that which is all around us. It was certainly true of our openness to receive input from the nursing staff in the past, indeed it is probably still true to a significant extent. I think it will become an increasing source of friction as we head into the 21st century and beyond and see computers get better and better at integrating complex information and consequently value human input less and less.

On a population basis, you see, computers are always going to do better than us at predicting outcomes. They have bigger numbers to run and can be constantly updating their database. Indeed, if we were to set up the system well, there could easily be a time where every primary care practitioner in every State of the Union is adding information moment by moment throughout their patient visits, alerting us to changing patterns of everything from infectious disease outbreaks to how much weight loss is associated with a specific intervention practice. Our role is not to try to assimilate all this data ourselves. It lies in providing a steadying hand to guide something that is inevitably protean and ungraspable. Let us, rather, look to the things that are representative of our real skill, the things that do not change with time or technology and which are not threatened by the vast computational power of electricity and gated potentials that encroaches all around.

At the heart of everything in medicine is the doctor patient interview and this is the one place that will remain challenging for computers to supersede their poor primate programmers. Here is the most important intersection in medical practice, the point at which we have to decide, "Is the person in front of me like everyone else or not?" What we must always be asking ourselves is, "Why is this person NOT the statistical average of the population? Why should I NOT to do what the computer says to do?" Because these are the moments when we transform medicine. This is when we add to the care of our patients and truly work in partnership with technology, making best use of all it has to offer without losing all that we have to contribute.

In order to do this we need as much information as possible about the individual in front of us. Not the lab tests; not the CAT scans. The personal history, the personal *story*. I think there are three big questions that eternally hover over the patient-health worker interaction. The first two questions are beguilingly simple: Who are you and what do you want? I was an actor for 20 years and I am acutely aware of the enormity of those questions. Plumbing the depths of a character for an answer to those two questions has been the essence of art for as long as our species has told stories to each other. Can we get anywhere near an answer in a 15 minute encounter? Of course not, but we have multiple inputs from people who spend many hours with them: nurses, physical therapists, social workers, chaplains, the list goes on. Each is a human interaction that will reveal a different detail to those that are sensitive enough to see. The lab tests will tell the computer the sum of the parts, but the body language and the light in the eyes will tell a story that is much deeper. Life is complex and the practice of medicine no less so. Our true skill is in this interpretation so that we will know how to evaluate the gambler's odds that the computer serves up to aid us.

Then, and only then, after we have come as close as we reasonably can to an understanding of who someone is and what they want, can we honestly ask the third and perhaps most difficult question, both for them and for us: "Can I help?" Because that involves doing what is best for them, not what is best for us and that may be a difficult place for us to see as well as a difficult place for us to go. To truly be stewards, we must strive to attain that knowledge and we need as many collaborators on that journey as we can muster. Hence, it behooves us to try to hold in the forefront of our minds the ideas that medicine is a team effort and that our number one job is to advocate for the patient. The one standing in front of us, not the one that is the total amalgam of the population he or she belongs to. If we keep that as our focus we will be in a good position to keep everything in the practice of medicine shipshape.

Questions

1. The author suggests looking to the past to see what has remained constant in the ever-changing field of medicine. What are some aspects of medicine that you feel will not or should not change?

2. How do you think William Osler's quote should affect medical education? How should it affect your clinical practice?

3. Can you think of a medical scenario in which the patient is not the statistical average and you should not do what the computer says to do?

—Roshini Selladurai

On Becoming a Doctor: Excellent Medical Student, Terrible Clinician

October 8, 2013

Amy Ho
University of Texas Southwestern Medical School
Class of 2014

T HERE IS A SAYING that you enter medical school wanting to help people but exit it wanting to help yourself. It may be a cynical view, but it is a realistic one. The criteria to being a good medical student are far different from being a good doctor. Medical education may be breeding a legion of self-serving, grade-grubbing, SOAP-note spewing machines rather than the "empathetic," "compassionate" and "caring" physicians of admissions essays yore.

I was no different. My first two years of medical school, I was largely a disinterested student; I didn't care for basic sciences, research or pathology. Like many others, my knowledge waxed and waned with the test schedule, and after Step 1, I entered my clinical years an acceptably successful medical student.

Excellent medical student, terrible clinician

Third year begins a reign of terror lead by the constant gauntlet of heavily-weighted rotation grades, standardized exams and the looming threat of residency applications and "The Match," when, after 20 years of schooling, some pie-in-the-sky computer would tell me if I was good enough or not to be a doctor, and subsequently determine my life for the next three to seven years.

Grades were a priority to make myself the most competitive residency candidate possible. I studied and worked hard. Each patient became an opportunity for me to impress on notes, rapid-fire oral presentations and predict nuanced "pimp" questions. I learned to charm patients just enough that they'd acknowledge my "care" to the attending during rounds. I interrogated my patients just enough to write the excellent notes I knew I'd be evaluated on. I "learned" about my patients by memorizing their daily lab values to proudly recite on rounds.

Patients weren't people with problems but stepping stones to rack up points with the attending. Once rounds were over, patients became time-sucks from shelf exam studying time, an exam worth 30% of every rotation grade. Real humans do not follow textbook presentations, but exams do; the warm body in front of me only detracted from my evaluation by cold Scantron. By my attendings' clinical comments, I was an "excellent medical student," but I knew I was a terrible clinician, rehearsed only in the games of academia, not medicine.

How I learned to stop worrying about The Match and love patient care

My shift in paradigm came with a shift in career path. My worst fear as a fledgling surgeon was not "matching" for a residency spot. My worst fear as a fledgling emergency physician was killing a patient. Suddenly playing doctor became very real, and in the middle of my OB/GYN rotation, I started to care not about textbook presentations but real-world ones. I didn't care for OB/GYN and volunteered to cover the peripartum critical care unit, a similar environment to emergency medicine.

My first day on the unit, I saw a patient roll in as I was in the middle of practice questions on the computer. I glanced up but returned to my test preparation, justifying my delay in evaluating the patient because the resident was still in surgery. Half an hour later, the resident came to evaluate the patient and I followed. The patient was obtunded, hypotensive and sitting in a growing pool of her own blood. It would not have taken a MD to realize that this patient required immediate medical attention, and I kicked myself for not evaluating her sooner. I may have been a pretend doctor, but it finally struck me that I was a pretend doctor on very real patients.

For the rest of my time in the unit, I made it a point to personally round every hour, on the hour, on every patient. I didn't always write notes for these hourly rounds; getting credit was no longer important to me, patient care was. While they initially questioned my obsessive rounding, the residents quickly came to trust my dedication and leave me to my own in the unit, knowing I'd alert them if necessary.

At my institution, hell hath no fury like an OB/GYN resident unnecessarily interrupted, so I spent my time reading on appropriate treatment courses for the different conditions I saw in the unit. After I rounded, I'd give the resident a list of orders to put in, and the nurses began to treat me as the main provider in the unit. I got to be the first person to make critical medical decisions, responding to truly acute situations and drastically changing the course of a patient's treatment. I pulled long hours and hardly studied in the traditional sense with prep books and practice questions, but I was constantly reading on my patients. That Shelf exam and clinical evaluations were my best of the year. I had learned to stop worrying about "The Match" and love patient care.

Not "just" a student

After that revelation, I fought to earn more responsibility and trust on each rotation; I learned more, gained competence and became more satisfied in my chosen career in medicine. During emergency medicine, the specialty that started it all for me, I learned more medicine in one month than I did in my entire third year. It was a pass/fail course with no motivation by grading, but I was terrified I would be the first person to evaluate a patient and not recognize a critical condition. That hemorrhaging patient from day one on the peripartum critical care unit still haunted me. People can decompensate quickly and unpredictably. At any moment, you may go from being "just" a student to being the only medical provider in the room.

At the end of that rotation, Step 2 breezed by with none of the misery I experienced with Step 1. Behind each question I'd see faces of patients with that exact presentation; behind each answer choice, I'd see the clinical consequence of making the wrong decision. Finally, I understood what it mean to be both an excellent medical student, and (at my level of training) an excellent clinician.

The academics of medicine often makes us forget the "59 yo AA M with pmh CHF dx 2010 (EF 20% by TTE 8/2013) p/w SOB x 2d" is a real person, with real vulnerabilities and real fears. We are not "just" students, but trainees and members of the medical profession. Grades and exams do not define us, but are simply checks on clinical competence. Trite as it may be, remember what you wrote about in your admissions essay: why you embarked on this journey in the first place. We came to medical school not to become excellent medical students, but to become excellent doctors. Always keep that in mind; all else, the grades, "The Match," the exams, will fall in place.

Questions

1. What experiences have played a role in transforming you from "just" a student into a clinician?

2. Have you ever felt like a "pretend doctor" during your training? How has this affected your approach to interacting with patients?

3. Do you feel that you are contributing to patient care in medical school? Why or why not?

4. In this narrative, the author speaks about patients as "stepping stones to rack up points." Do you ever feel this way? What strategies have you used to treat patients as people? How do you plan to hold onto your humanity throughout your training and beyond?

—Aleena Paul

A Letter to Myself, Future Resident, on Dealing with Myself, Current Medical Student

May 5, 2014

Lindsay Heuser
University of Colorado Denver School of Medicine
Class of 2015

DEAR (FUTURE) SELF,

I imagine that you're busy right now. Like really busy. Like the coffee-driven, adrenaline-fueled, sleep-deprived kind of busy that you experienced to a lesser degree in medical school except now you're actually expected to care for patients. Of course, by "care for patients," I mean "avoid doing dumb things to patients." A terrifying thought, the burden of patient care, but I'm sure you're learning and becoming more confident by the day. Why, you're becoming a real physician now! No longer do you float around the hospital following the residents around like a duckling, attempting to show that you too can think independently and provide assessments and plans like a good medical student. No, you are the resident now. The follower has become the followed. You are the mama duck.

And so, self, I am here writing to you as a current medical student on appropriate ways to deal with these so-called ducklings. It seems to me that the vast majority of residents tend to forget what it once was like to be a duckling. How it felt to desperately yearn to have actual responsibility over patients or to be constantly, actively thinking about each and every patient problem because it hasn't yet become automatic. The algorithms that physicians instantly zip through in their head run a little (okay, a lot) slower in these duckling students. I know they run a little slower in my head now, but with time and practice, these things will become automatic, as I imagine they are for you and most residents. I would like to think that you're self-aware enough to remember a time when you struggled with the great transformation from didactic thinking to clinical thinking and are thus gentle to any student in the midst of the learning process. But just as a reminder, here are a handful of tips, as selected by your younger self, a current medical

334

student, to better handle any medical students you may encounter during the resident journey:

1. Make a valiant effort to let the medical student interview the patient first. Remember how much you once hated shadowing? Well, it still stinks. Try to let students interview the patient first, present to you, and remind them that it's okay if they don't have the correct assessment and plan as long as they try to put one out there. Of course, to even have the opportunity to provide an assessment and plan, the student has to interview the patient first. It's pretty much a requirement. Remember, independent thinking starts with independent doing.

2. Medical students *love* to be helpful. Now, this doesn't mean make medical students do dumb tasks like retrieving coffee. It means, give them useful tasks that simultaneously help you out with your workload. Have them communicate updates to patients and their families. Let them have a first stab at writing the history and physical. Encourage them to take responsibility over the patients assigned to them. Giving medical students some semblance of structure and accountability makes their little hearts soar. Whatever you do, just don't ignore them. Few things in the world are sadder than a medical student scorned.

3. Let the medical student free at the end of the day. Remember how awful it was when you had nothing to do, and you were trapped in the hospital because your resident hadn't given you the "okay" to leave at the end of the day? Often, medical students express their desire to go home with the age-old question, "Is there anything else I can help you with?" You know you asked this question *many* times. When your students ask you this, and there truly is nothing for them to do, set them free. In fact, if there's nothing for them to do, be proactive and release them before they even ask you the question. This goes back to the idea of acknowledging the presence of a student on your team. Medical students have certain limitations because they are, well, medical students. If the work left for the day can only be done by a resident, be merciful on the student, and send them away from the hospital to study, eat, sleep, see friends and family, etcetera. While you may have longer hours as a resident, students have the additional obligation of studying for shelf exams and other such delights outside of their time at the hospital. Remember when that was you? Let them do this studying (and/or life living) on their own at home in the peace of a location that is not the hospital.

4. Be patient when a student has a brain fart. It's happened to you. It's happened to all of us. Those times when an attending asks a question that you know and then poof...the answer flits away from your head, only to return after you have stared blank-faced at the attending for several seconds. Thoughts are racing through your head. So much is happening up there, and yet, only an "uhhhh..." has departed from your lips. Smile at them when this happens, and remind them that it's "okay" if they don't know the answer today. Encourage them to learn it for tomorrow, and give them more than just a single chance to succeed.

5. Above all, know that you can make an impact on a medical student, even if they're on your service for only a day. The best residents you encountered during medical school were the ones that went above and beyond in their effort to teach you. They asked you what you wanted to get out of the rotation and tailored their teaching to your interests. Those residents were the ones that stuck out, and for all the best reasons. They were sincere, passionate educators. You can be like them too. You just need to make it a priority to take each student's education seriously. Don't buy into the excuse that a student needs to be on your service for a month before you'll incorporate them into the team. Don't buy into the excuse that you're too busy to educate medical students. Don't buy into cynicism in general. Embrace each new student on your service regardless of how long they'll be with you, and do your best to teach the heck out of your specialty. All you need is a day to make an impact.

And so, self, I think most of my advice to you, the resident, on dealing with medical students harkens back to the adage of "Remember where you once came from." We were all learners at one point or another. We struggled, we goofed up and we endured. Never ever forget that you were once the person struggling in front of you. That you once lacked the innate confidence and instinctual knowledge you now possess. Teach your students when you have free time. Make sure they know the team's lunch plans for the day. Give them advice on where to park and when to show up. Make them look good in front of attendings. Don't make them feel awkward if they come dangerously close to following you into the restroom. Be the best mama duck that you can be, and treat those ducklings with grace, finesse and kindness. I know you can do it during your residency and beyond.

Love,
Your (younger) self

Questions

1. Every resident was first a medical student. Why do you think residents and faculty forget what it was like to be a medical student?

2. What do you think will be the most difficult part of transitioning from a medical student to a resident?

3. What might you do if you or a classmate is not being treated well by a resident?

4. Have you had a resident who has been a particularly good role model and mentor? In what ways? Will you strive to emulate this resident when you are a resident yourself?

—Chelcie Soroka

"Are There Any Physicians on Board, We Have a Medical Emergency"

July 8, 2014

Manik Aggarwal
Texas A&M Health Science Center College of Medicine
Class of 2014

"DR. AGGARWAL, SHOULD WE divert the plane towards Salt Lake City? *Dr. Aggarwal*, Dr. Aggarwal, do you want to land in Salt Lake City?"

Until this point, it was always "Manik," and it was a basic question. If I was right, my intern or resident would be enthused with my knowledge; if I was wrong, they would teach and talk me up to rebuild my confidence. Well, that was last month.

This month, it's no longer Manik Aggarwal, MS4, and it's certainly no longer enthusiasm versus an opportunity for didactics. Now, it's Dr. Manik Aggarwal, MD, with a critical question to be answered urgently and an acutely sick patient at the bedside (err, in the airplane aisle).

As I left Portland that morning to get back home to Dallas, my best friend and I chatted all weekend about starting residency in the coming weeks. I did not realize that my first true test was moments away.

As I sat in the window seat of the exit row, I saw her stand up, grab her belly, and begin grimacing in an "impending doom" kind of way. She took a few steps in the aisle and collapsed. She literally crumbled to her knees. Without much thought or rationale at the time, I jumped over to help her. She was mostly non-responsive and had a very weak radial pulse, with a mild carotid pulse. She was mumbling her words and having a hard time staying alert. Then, those daunted and gut-wrenching words were spoken over the PA system: "We have a medical emergency. Are there any physicians on board?" Although I rejoiced in this call to my fellow colleagues, apparently none of them were on the plane to join me. With the help of outstanding crew members, I was able to sit the passenger-turned-patient upright.

As she began to mumble her words with slightly more clarity, she was able to deny chest pain and shortness of breath, but specifically said, "My belly started hurting just now and it's going up to my chest, and I vomited and have had diarrhea for three days now." This was followed by her then going pulseless and falling limp in seat 21F. Just like I learned in "The House of God" the prior week, before going into a code, check your own pulse. Thankfully mine was still ticking and we quickly went to work.

This was the moment that those words will forever be with me: "Dr. Aggarwal, do you want to divert to Salt Lake City?"

We attached an AED with fear she may be having an MI or another acute cardiac event that could lead to a potentially fatal arrhythmia. Much to our relief, she was sinus with a fluctuating but present pulse. With her benign past medical history and current history with signs and symptoms of dehydration, I administered water orally. Unfortunately, she vomited out the water and began fluctuating in consciousness again. At this point, I requested an IV kit with the basic assumption that if successful, she would perk right up, but if unsuccessful, we would be descending into Salt Lake City. Much to our excitement and relief, the IV was started successfully and normal saline flowed rapidly.

As expected with hypovolemia secondary to dehydration, she responded appropriately to the IV fluids and quickly began to perk up. There was no Salt Lake City, but there was a very anxious Dr. Aggarwal sitting in 21E the remainder of the flight.

As we began to descend into Dallas, the patient was chatting like normal and she politely asked out of partial fear, "So you look awfully young ... when did you finish your medical training?" Squeamishly, I suggested she wait for my answer until we land on ground before possibly sending her into shock again! With encouragement from her, I gulped and told her, "I walked across the stage during medical school graduation ten days ago ... you are my first patient."

Sharing this story with levity is fun and easy because we are all thankful that she did well. As a message to my medical students reading this: keep in mind that you're learning pathophysiology to take care of a sick human being. Will better grades or board scores be a byproduct? Yes. Will getting into the residency of your choice serve as the ultimate sign of success? Yes. But, before you know it, it may be your ultimate decision to make. So, Future Doctor, are we diverting to Salt Lake City?

Questions

1. How would you react to this situation, being a recent graduate and the only health care provider on the flight?

2. How do stories like this help us keep perspective on future patients while we study pathophysiology?

3. The author points out that he readily shared this story because the outcome was positive. Do you think we should share stories where the outcome is not positive? Why or why not?

4. Why do you think it is important to check your own pulse before jumping into an emergency?

—Melanie Watt

Is It Better to Trust or to Hope?

March 17, 2015

Robert Ethel
University of Oklahoma College of Medicine
Class of 2016

S INCE THE START OF my third year as a medical student, I have been quite interested in observing how people interact with me now that I am wearing a white coat. To be more specific, I find it amazing that people do not realize that my white coat is so much shorter than everyone else's. To me, the length of my coat should act as a warning to those around me; I do not know where things are, and I do not know what's going on most of the time. It is this white coat however, which instantaneously turns me into a well-trusted and well-respected member of society.

Even before entering medical school, I was quite aware that society holds physicians in high regard. My recent experiences, however, have forced me to ask, "Why do a certain subpopulation of people, almost blindly, trust and believe what doctors say and do?"

I know that doctors make mistakes (although our training aims to eliminate much wrong-doing) and do not always act appropriately. Therefore, it is hard to understand from where this blind trust is drawn. Taking a careful look at the patients and their physicians around me, I have come to the belief that this trust goes beyond our simple definition of trust. I argue that there is something else driving this sometimes blind trust that patients have in their physicians, and that the very thing creating this driving force is the advancement of modern day medicine itself.

According to a Gallup Health and Healthcare Survey in 2010 of 511 adults age 18 and over, 70 percent of Americans are confident in their doctor's advice and do not feel a need to seek out a second opinion or do additional research on their own. But what does it mean for patients to trust in their physician? What is this trust composed of?

Trust can be defined as a belief that someone is good, honest and reliable. So how is a physician good, honest and reliable? Of note, a physician's extensive training and knowledge in diagnosing and treating medical conditions within their field creates a system in which patients must rely on the expertise of their physicians. Additionally, physicians are trained to empathize with patients, respect patient autonomy, and make ethically sound decisions when it comes to a patient's health. The profession itself expects a certain standard for physicians to be caring, honest, knowledgeable, and reliable when determining health care decisions for patients. Thus, a certain level of training, standards and professional expectations merge to create an ethically good, honest, and medically reliable individual — the physician — in whom patients can place their trust. But how is this trust different from other types of trust that people place in professionals? If we take the aforementioned definition of trust, we can simply apply it to many circumstances. For example, people trust their mechanic to fix their car properly. People also trust their dentist to take care of their teeth properly. They trust them because they believe that they have a certain skill set which can reliably fix a problem, and that they will do so in a good and honest way. However, the trust that I see in the hospital from some patients is different from the trust they put in their mechanic; this trust goes beyond the simple definition of trust previously addressed.

I have noted on the floors that there is a subset of patients who believe their physician is more than just good, honest and reliable. There is something else in the mind of the patient when the doctor is explaining the diagnosis and treatment for their cancer. I believe that this something else is hope. Hope that their physician will cure them and get them feeling better. Hope that their cancer will be eradicated. Hope that they will once again resume their daily lives with their families.

If trust comes from a belief that a person is good, honest and reliable, then where does a patient's hope come from? I believe this hope comes from a belief in the power of medicine. Patients believe that the power of modern day medicine will work for them, and this creates hope. When patients hear that they have cancer, some react with fear, but for others, their initial reaction is one of hope. They cling to every word as the doctors explain advanced medical treatments, hopeful that a medical miracle lies somewhere in those words.

They believe that the all-powerful modern day medicine can help them. They may have heard or read about Gleevec, the cancer-killing wonder pill that melts away cancer in months. They may have heard of medical advancements in everything from antibiotics, to radical life-saving surgical procedures, to finding and destroying cancers with MRI and proton therapy machines. Due to medicine's continued efficacy and progress, and for some patients, a lack of comprehension, many in society have developed a belief in the healing power of medicine.

It is a belief that Medicine (with a capital M) can cure everything — a belief that Medicine will beat AIDS, that Medicine will cure cancer, and that Medicine will allow our children to live longer than us. For some, medicine has been elevated beyond pure physiology and biological facts to an otherworldly belief in its efficacy. For some, Medicine is analogous to magic — with physicians being the revered wielders of that magic. When a patient's hope in the healing power of medicine emerges, and combines with their trust in a physician, the patient looks at the physician through a different pair of eyes. Patients at times do more than merely "trust" physicians with their health care: they revere them, in the hope that they may lay their healing hands upon them and employ the magic that is modern day Medicine to heal them of their ills.

So, if hope is present in the minds of some patients when they interact with physicians, what does this mean for how they make health care decisions? How does this affect the patient-physician relationship? When one thinks of hope, it is mostly thought of in a positive light. Hope can give patients motivation and a will to fight harder. Unfortunately, recent events show that while the power of medicine brings hope, complacency is not too far behind.

When the power of medicine is looked upon through the lens of the sick, it prevailingly produces hope, hope that the power of medicine will cure. But, when the power of medicine is gazed upon through the lens of the healthy, it can produce complacency. Take for example, the anti-vaccination movement. If parents believe that modern medicine can tackle any disease, including those diseases which their children are routinely vaccinated against, parents are led down the path of opting out of giving vaccines to their children. If the rare disease that could potentially hurt a child can be effectively treated by modern medicine, and there remains some perceived risk involved with the vaccine, it is not difficult to see how parents make what they believe is the logical conclusion to opt out of the vaccine.

Yet another example of how hope can lead to complacency is noncompliance by patients in the care of their chronic diseases such as hypertension and diabetes. Hypertension and diabetes both do not make the patient feel "sick." The patient may be warned about the consequences of noncompliance of their chronic disease but if there is a belief in the all-powerful efficacy of medicine to cure any consequence that may arise, there will be less motivation for patients to manage their disease appropriately when they are feeling "fine."

The dangerous aspect of the power of medicine comes from society's general misunderstanding of it. Patients may not understand that measles is a terrible disease and difficult to manage, even with modern medicine. Patients may not understand that very little can be done for a non-compliant diabetic patient with multiple diabetic ulcers and end-stage kidney disease. Patients may not understand that chemotherapy and radiation may only extend the life of a stage 4 cancer patient by one month. The list goes on and on. All patients hear about is how modern medicine cured this and made that patient's life better — and even with all the malpractice commercials and questioning of physicians, the medical miracles are what some patients choose to hear and remember. For some, medicine has been elevated beyond evaluation, diagnosis, and treatment to a revered belief in its efficacy.

The last point that I believe warrants discussion is how the aforementioned hope alters the patient-physician relationship. When this hope is factored in, it creates a mindset in the patient that is different than if they merely trusted their physician. As future physicians, we need to be cognizant of the power of this hope in some patients. Patient autonomy is often quickly tossed aside in lieu of a patient's hope in medicine. When a complicated surgical procedure is explained to a patient, they are not comforted by the biological and anatomical aspects of the surgery, or the fact that the drug targets the HER2 receptors on their breast cancer cells. They trust in the physician and, maybe more importantly, are hopeful that the great and powerful Medicine can cure them. So, they defer to the all-powerful doctor to do whatever it is that they do to produce medical miracles. In doing so, the patient is handing over their autonomy and picking up some hope from the promise of Medicine.

As science continues to progress, become more complex, and produce more medical miracles, this hope in the efficacy of medicine will only grow, leading to further deferment of patient autonomy to the physician. Eventually, will the hope that modern medicine provides to patients drown out their trust in the physician? Will patients allow doctors to take full control of their health care due the complexity of the treatments and the patient's hope that it will work? There are questions that must be present in the minds of future physicians as we progress through our training in order to fully care for a patient — not only medically, but psychologically and emotionally as well.

Questions

1. Since starting medical school, have you noticed people treating you differently?

2. How should a physician balance trust and hope when delivering bad news to a patient?

3. How do physicians ensure patients don't develop false hope?

4. How can we explain the complexities of medicine to patients in ways that do not promote blind faith?

—Roshini Selladurai

References

Medical Student, Student Physician or Student Doctor?
1. Lemert C, Branaman A. *The Goffman Reader.* Cambridge, MA: Wiley Blackwell Readers, 1997. Print.
2. Park RE. *Race and Culture.* Glencoe, IL: Free Press, 1950. Print.
3. Kleinman A. *The Illness Narratives: Suffering, Healing, and the Human Condition.* New York, NY: Basic Books, 1988. Print.
4. Marracino RK, Orr RD. Entitling the student doctor: defining the student's role in patient care. *J Gen Intern Med.* 1998 Apr;13(4):266-70.
5. Griffin M, Block JW. *In the Company of the Poor: Conversations with Dr. Paul Farmer and Fr. Gustavo Gutiérrez.* Orbis Books, 2013. Print.

Treating the Disease and Treating the Illness
1. Wolpert L. *Six Impossible Things before Breakfast: The Evolutionary Origins of Belief.* New York, NY: W.W. Norton & Company, 2006. Print.
2. Pinker S. *The Stuff of Thought: Language as a Window into Human Nature.* New York, NY: Penguin, 2007. Print.

A Lack of Care: Why Medical Students Should Focus on Ferguson
1. Todd KH, et al. Ethnicity and analgesic practice. *Ann Emerg Med.* 2000 Jan;35(1):11-6.
2. McNeil CB, et al. Cultural issues in the treatment of young African American children diagnosed with disruptive behavior disorders. *J Pediatr Psychol.* 2002;27(4):339-50.
3. Crystal S, et al. Broadened use of atypical antipsychotics: safety, effectiveness, and policy challenges. *Health Aff.* 2009 Sep-Oct;28(5):w770-81.
4. Tamayo-Sarver JH, et al. Racial and ethnic disparities in emergency department analgesic prescription. *Am J Public Health.* 2003 Dec;93(12):2067-73.
5. Knafo S. "When It Comes To Illegal Drug Use, White America Does The Crime, Black America Gets The Time." *The Huffington Post.* 17 Sept. 2013.
6. New York Civil Liberties Union (NYCLU). "Stop-and-Frisk Data." American Civil Liberties Union of New York State. Retrieved 1 Dec. 2014. http://www.nyclu.org/content/stop-and-frisk-data.
7. Braun L. Race, ethnicity, and health: can genetics explain disparities? *Perspect Biol Med.* 2002 Spring;45(2):159-74.
8. Satcher D, et al. What if we were equal? A comparison of the black-white mortality gap in 1960 and 2000. *Health Aff.* 2005 Mar-Apr;24(2):459-64.
9. Fang J, et al. The association between birthplace and mortality from cardiovascular causes among black and white residents of New York City. *N Engl J Med.* 1996 Nov 21;335(21):1545-51.
10. Higgins RS, et al. Disparities in solid organ transplantation for ethnic minorities: facts and solutions. *Am J Transplant.* 2006 Nov;6(11):2556-62.
11. Sack K. "Research Finds Wide Disparities in Health Care by Race and Region." *The New York Times.* 5 June 2008.
12. Gornick ME, et al. Effects of race and income on mortality and use of services among Medicare beneficiaries. *N Engl J Med.* 1996 Sep 12;335(11):791-9.

Physicians-in-Transit: The Blizzard of 2015
1. Bebinger M. "Listen: How Health Care Facilities Are Preparing For The Blizzard." *CommonHealth*. WBUR. 26 Jan. 2015.
2. Phelps J. "Region's Hospitals Gear up for the Storm." *MetroWest Daily News*. 27 Jan. 2015.
3. Lacy NL, et al. Why we don't come: patient perceptions on no-shows. *Ann Fam Med*. 2004 Nov-Dec;2(6):541-5.
4. Green AR, et al. Barriers to screening colonoscopy for low-income Latino and white patients in an urban community health center. *J Gen Intern Med*. 2008 Jun;23(6):834–40.
5. Tait AR, et al. Cancellation of pediatric outpatient surgery: economic and emotional implications for patients and their families. *J Clin Anesth*. 1997 May;9(3):213-9.
6. Marcus AC, et al. Improving adherence to screening follow-up among women with abnormal Pap smears: results from a large clinic-based trial of three intervention strategies. *Med Care*. 1992 Mar;30(3):216-30.

On Silence: The Limits of Professionalism
1. Lorde A. *The Cancer Journals*. San Francisco, CA: Aunt Lute Books, 1997. Print.
2. Ainsworth-Vaughn N. *Claiming Power in Doctor-Patient Talk*. New York, NY: Oxford University Press, 1998. Print.
3. Salinger T. "Sigma Alpha Epsilon Closes Okla. Chapter over Racist Video." *New York Daily News*. 25 Mar. 2015.

Do You Remember?
1. Goldman B. "Brian Goldman: Doctors Make Mistakes. Can We Talk about That?" YouTube. TED, 25 Jan. 2012. http://www.youtube.com/watch?v=iUbfRzxNy20.

Fading Memories of Love and Martinis
1. Kleinman A. *What Really Matters: Living a Moral Life Amidst Uncertainty and Danger*. New York, NY: Oxford University Press, 2006. Print.
2. Stoppard T. *Rosencrantz and Guildenstern Are Dead*. London: Faber and Faber, 1968. Print.

A Case for Inclusive Language
1. Balasubramanian J. "Do No Harm: Queer Patients and the Med School Closet." *Fusion*. 16 Mar. 2015.
2. Pololi LH, et al. Experiencing the culture of academic medicine: gender matters, a national study. *J Gen Intern Med*. 2013 Feb;28(2):201-7.
3. Beagan BL. 'Is this worth getting into a big fuss over?' Everyday racism in medical school. *Med Educ*. 2003 Oct;37(10):852-60.
4. Marques AM, et al. Lesbians on medical encounters: tales of heteronormativity, deception, and expectations. *Health Care Women Int*. 2015 Sep;36(9):988-1006.

Wounded Healers

1. American Foundation for Suicide Prevention (AFSP). "Physician and Medical Student Depression and Suicide Prevention." Retrieved 1 Nov. 2014. http://afsp.org/our-work/education/physician-medical-student-depression-suicide-prevention.

2. Goebert D, et al. Depressive symptoms in medical students and residents: a multischool study. *Acad Med.* 2009 Feb;84(2):236-41.

3. Drake D. "How Being a Doctor Became the Most Miserable Profession." *The Daily Beast.* 14 Apr. 2014.

4. Levine RE, et al. The depressed physician: a different kind of impairment. *Hospital Physician.* 2000 Feb;67-73.

5. Dyrbye LN, et al. Relationship between burnout and professional conduct and attitudes among US medical students. *JAMA.* 2010 Sep 15;304(11):1173-80.

6. Zoccolillo M, et al. Depression among medical students. *J Affect Disord.* 1986 Jul-Aug;11(1):91-6.

7. Vaillant GE, et al. Some psychologic vulnerabilities of physicians. *N Engl J Med.* 1972 Aug 24;287(8):372-5.

8. Johnson WD. Predisposition to emotional distress and psychiatric illness amongst doctors: the role of unconscious and experiential factors. *Br J Med Psychol.* 1991 Dec;64(Pt 4):317-29.

9. Ely E. "From Bipolar Darkness, the Empathy to Be a Doctor." *The New York Times.* 16 Apr. 2009.

10. Feldman MD, et al. Let's not talk about it: suicide inquiry in primary care. *Ann Fam Med.* 2007 Sep-Oct;5(5):412-8.

11. Center C, et al. Confronting depression and suicide in physicians: a consensus statement. *JAMA.* 2003 Jun 18;289(23):3161-6.

12. Schwenk TL, et al. Depression, stigma, and suicidal ideation in medical students. *JAMA.* 2010 Sep 15;304(11):1181-90.

13. Elkins R. *My Bright Shining Star: A Mother's True Story of Brilliance, Love & Suicide.* Perfect Publishers Ltd., 2014. Print.

14. Elkins R. "My Bright Shining Star." Retrieved 1 Nov. 2014. http://welding81.wordpress.com.

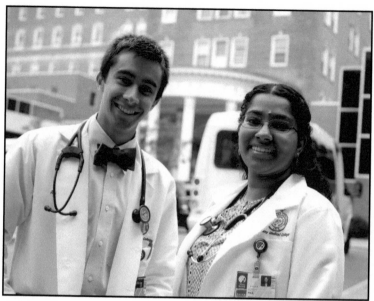

Ajay and Aleena met at Union College in Schenectady, New York in 2008 as students in the Leadership in Medicine Program. They both joined the student newspaper, the *Concordiensis*, and became fast friends after countless hours of newspaper editing, Bollywood songs and late-night coffee runs.

Motivated by their business training at Union Graduate College, Ajay and Aleena decided to continue their work in journalism by founding *in-Training* in April 2012, just prior to matriculating at Albany Medical College. Four years and hundreds of articles later, Ajay and Aleena have finally brought their a dream to life: a print compendium of medical student voices, *in-Training: Stories from Tomorrow's Physicians*.

When not working on *in-Training*, Ajay is a student advocate focused on empowering medical students to become change agents in medicine through the written word and social media. He is also an avid reader of all things sci-fi and fantasy. Aleena is a national leader with the American Medical Women's Association (AMWA) with an emphasis on mentoring future leaders in medicine. She is also working on her watercolor painting and pottery skills.

Ajay will be starting his residency in internal medicine at the University of Colorado School of Medicine and Aleena will be starting her residency in internal medicine-pediatrics at the University of Massachusetts School of Medicine.